MAKE YOUR FACE YOUR FORTUNE

*a top makeup artist shows you how to make
the exact beauty & personality statement you want, for any occasion*

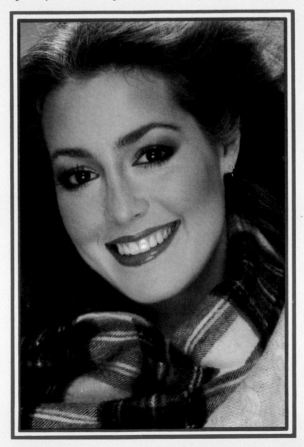

PETER SHEN with JOYCE WILSON

originally published as *Peter Shen's Makeup for Success*

Make Your Face
Your Fortune

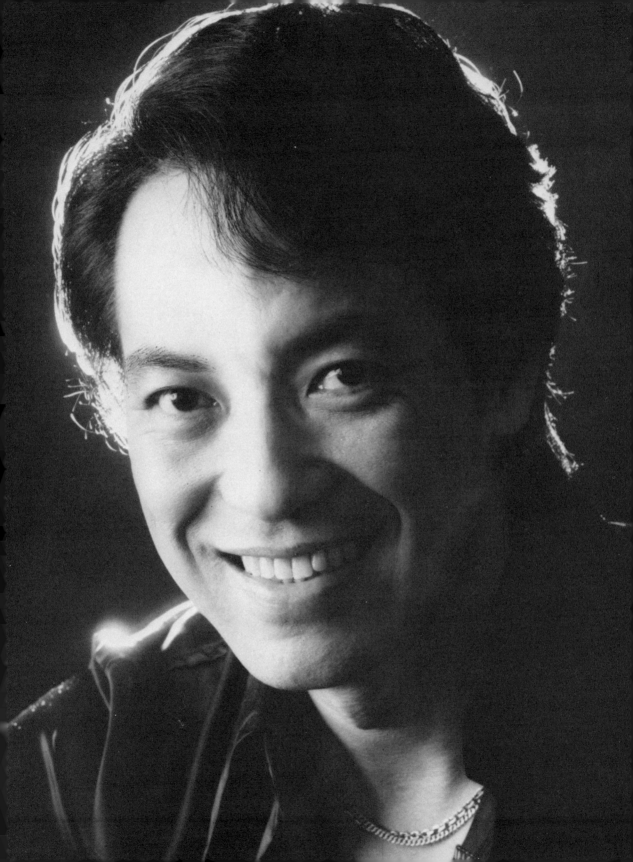

Make Your Face Your Fortune

by Peter Shen with Joyce Wilson

EVEREST HOUSE Publishers, New York

LIBRARY OF CONGRESS CATALOGING IN PUBLICATION DATA:

Shen, Peter, 1939–
  Make your face your fortune.

  Originally published: Peter Shen's Makeup for success.
1st ed. New York, Everest House, c. 1980.
  1. Beauty, Personal.   2. Cosmetics.   3. Physiognomy.
I. Milo, Mary, 1915–   . II. Title.
RA778.S55   1982   646.7'26   82-11431
ISBN: 0-89696-075-7
      0-89696-181-8 (pbk.)

Published by Everest House,
33 West 60th Street, New York, N.Y. 10023
Published simultaneously in Canada by
Beaverbooks, Don Mills, Ontario
Manufactured in the United States of America
Designed by Joyce Cameron Weston
RRD882

Contents

What This Book Can Do for You

YES—"YOUR FACE IS YOUR FORTUNE." The ancient Chinese put it this way: "Beauty is destiny." Here for the first time are efficient makeup techniques for busy women—the working woman, home-maker, student, businesswoman, professional—combined with simple and interesting ways to learn the basic art of Face Reading. According to Face Reading, who you are, what you are like and what you can do is written on your face.

Here you can learn what each feature represents and how you can modify it or emphasize it to become more accessible to what you de-sire—a more contented marriage, a happier love relationship, a better job, success, fame, fortune, or even just a more gratifying day-to-day experience. For example:

- Do you know why overheavy brows—or too thin brows—can be off-putting? (The first are too callous; the second, too self-indul-gent.)

- Have you ever considered the meaning of the groove between the nose and upper lip that helps form a cupid's bow? (It's sexy!)

- Is it possible your nose can make you rich—just as it is? Find out before you have a nose job.

- Choosing a mate? Will he be generous or stingy? His ears will tell. Will he be true or philandering? Look at his lips—and count the crinkles at the corners of his eyes.

You can discover these and other personality pointers and learn much more about your own face—and others' faces—by studying the Map of the Face, its Three Stations, its Five Major Features and Seven

Minor Features—along with clues from complexion color, hair, and even teeth. And the more you know about the meaning of your features, the more cleverly you can make up your face.

Most women make up their face with little or no idea of what they are trying to *say*. This is a beauty guide that tells you exactly what you need to do to your eyebrows, your mouth, your hair—and why. People who look at you, those who are going to offer you a job, a promotion, a business opportunity, or who are going to invite you on an important first date or to a party, probably aren't going to know a thing about face and feature reading (unless they've also read this book). But they are subliminally going to take in what your face says about you. Your basic face tells a lot; your makeup tells even more.

Here are ways to understand your face and to use makeup to say what you want to say about yourself. You can make a better impression once you know what *is* impressive in the color, shape, and prominence of a feature, and how to use makeup to express the positive.

You will find out how to use makeup and other cosmetic arts to change your looks for the better—even the best—and help your life become remarkable, not just plain dull.

You'll discover how makeup can lead not only to better looks but to fame and fortune and success and above all to harmony between your inner self and the outer world.

No beauty book has ever been able to offer so much self-confidence.

WHAT IS FACE READING?

The Chinese art of Face Reading—physiognomy—goes back to the time of Confucius in the fifth century B.C., the spring and autumn periods of Chinese culture. Later, during the Chin and Han periods, the analysis of the Points on the Map of the Face (see page 18) were put into verses and the face reader would recite the relevant rhymes as he studied the face of the one who came for a reading. Since this time, several traditions of Face Reading have developed. In this book we follow the ancient teaching of a school called the "Linen Robe."

Face Reading is actually character reading, not divination. That is, it defines your aptitudes, talents and capacities, but does not reveal the future, except insofar as your destiny depends on your natural endowments and upon the condition of the areas of the face concerned with your goals. What you do with your inborn characteristics is up to you.

Understanding what these capacities are will help you make the most of your looks, your personality, your life.

FACE AND FEATURE READING—WHY RELEVANT TO MAKEUP?

Why is the art of face and feature reading so important a part of makeup? Simply because your makeup is a statement of your role as a woman. Actors and actresses have always understood this. Stage or screen makeup is different if one plays an empress, a business-woman, a woman detective, a playgirl, a student, a homemaker—because this is the quickest way for a player to establish identity in her role. But the way actresses make up for the screen has also defined the changing role of women in our society. This is easy to understand if you look back at the change in screen makeup in the past several decades. Anyone can do this today because so many old movies are being shown on television.

Let's remember that the use of makeup by women generally came in only with the movies—and makeup techniques have developed right along with the motion pictures and television.

In the very early days of the silent movies, the heroines—Mary Pickford, Billie Burke, the Gish sisters, Pearl White—always had droopy eyebrows and little round mouths, because these are the signs of dependency in women, and women then were expected to be dependent upon men. As the glamorous worldly women took over in the 1930s—Marlene Dietrich, Greta Garbo, Jean Harlow, for example—the thin highly arched brows and wider sensuous mouth became the fashion to emphasize the sophistication that women were achieving.

During World War II, when women had to rely more on themselves, the straight ''career-woman'' eyebrows and matte well-formed mouth were the keynote (Greer Garson, Irene Dunne), while the pinups played up their sensuous mouths and full eyes but still with stronger brows.

After the war, when women went back to the home to have babies, there was a more innocent look again—Marilyn Monroe (even though a sex symbol) had a childlike innocence. But then the *strong-woman* actresses of that period—Sophia Loren, for example—brought in the extended, heavily lined eyes and knife-shaped brows of the adventuress.

After that we experienced a totally natural, almost childlike "bareface" look and the offbeat looks of the hippy period.

Only now, when the social structure is for very individualized roles for women, do we see the return of the smoother, more precise look in makeup. Women today look "experienced" and self-possessed —and they have enough skill with makeup and enough fine cosmetics available to shape their features and face for the look that will interpret for them whichever of the various roles they may choose to play.

With so many women choosing to make their way in a career, the brow and eye areas have become particularly important—because they represent fame, achievement, and equal status in society. Each woman, like an actress on the screen, is defining her role with her makeup to command the attention and respect she deserves,

The better you understand the meaning of features and the areas of the face, the better you can interpret your own role.

This book gets you off to a good start both as a face reader and makeup expert. But become a face watcher too. Observe what people in the movies, on television, in magazines are like and what they do with their makeup to conceal and reveal their personality and character. You will discover much about what you can do with your own face.

Make Your Face Your Fortune

1. How to Read the Map of the Face

WHAT DO YOU LOOK for when you read the Map of the Face? Each of the numbered points on the map—Position Points—represents a year in the life, beginning with the time of birth—Point 1—and going around the ears, forehead, eyes, nose, mouth, cheeks, chin, and hairline to Point 100 (completion) under the chin.

The point that represents your current age is most indicative of your present life circumstances. There will be a slight glow around this Position Point if you are to have a happy healthy rewarding year. If the glow isn't there now, you can help it become apparent.

Other Position Points and Palaces (significant areas of the face) will enter into your understanding of what in life is at present affecting you. For example, the area under your lower lip, if it is full and robust, indicates you will travel comfortably; the triangles above the outer tip of the brows also are "motion" areas. If you plan a trip and these areas are pink and glowing, the trip will be advantageous. There are "promotion points" that indicate a rise in position; "society" points that indicate charm, and so on around the entire face.

The face is also seen as composed of mountains and rivers. The mouth, eyes and nostrils—features that produce moisture—are the rivers; the high points—forehead, chin, nose and cheekbones—are the mountains. Like a country, you need a balanced terrain. For example, a large nose in an otherwise flat face—a mountain unsupported by other prominences—is not considered fortunate. A flat nose surrounded by other prominent features may mean you have to work hard all your life.

Areas of the face have distinctive lucky colors. If the nose has a golden glow, it indicates success in a venture. Purplish color between the eyes indicates a promotion.

Do you have moles on your face? If so, you probably have another mole on a corresponding part of your body. Generally, exposed moles (on your face) are not considered lucky; hidden moles are lucky. Some facial moles, though, are beneficial. A mole on the cheek at the "society point" (in the dimple area) indicates social success, chattiness, charm—but it is considered negative for marriage.

To read the map of the face, you have to consider the whole face—the Position Points, the Three Stations, the Five Major Features, the Seven Minor Features, the shape of the head and face and even their size and how the various features balance or cancel one another out.

If you are considering someone as a sexual partner for example—or evaluating your own potential charm—you would look at the age point to be sure it is warm and glowy, and for at least a few of the following characteristics:

· Light eyebrows with loose hairs
· Deep laugh lines
· Large mouth with full lips
· Full—even protruding—eyes
· High cheekbones
· Deep groove between the nostrils and the upper lip
· Protruding ears
· An upturned "pug nose" or a nose that points down
· Strong chin
· Circles under the eyes
· A tendency to keep the mouth open
· Thick hair
· Deep voice
· Large head
· Freckles
· Brows highly arched
· Laugh crinkles at the corners of the eyes (in a man, especially)

Anyone may have one or two of these characteristics, of course, and few have them all. Someone who shows a great many of them may prove to be overly sexually indulgent. Along with their presence, you should evaluate their quality. Is the groove from the nostrils to the upper lip flared at the bottom or top or is it straight? Are the ears large or small, set high or low on the head? Is the nose large or tight through the bridge? Do you or your prospective partner have a horizontal line between the brows? In a man, this means he is hard on his mate and family.

Freckles, protruding ears, a pug nose—sexy? It's clear that it isn't always the beautiful features that make us attractive.

The oval face, the so-called ideal face for beauty, though an asset in youth, is not promising for long life or robust health in the later years. And the ideal nose—small, straight, narrow—goes against happiness in marriage.

In looking for a mate, you would also want to know whether he is likely to be wealthy or a hard worker or a spendthrift. How long will he live? What are his career chances?

Luckily, most of us have some good features—good for success, relationships, health, vitality, attractiveness—along with the poor features that create problems to overcome, just as we each have at least one good feature for beauty. Obviously, those features favorable for fortune and those favorable for beauty are not always the same.

Some people are even lucky enough to have five poor features. Lucky? Yes. If the Five Major Features are bad, it somehow turns your luck around, and brings you success. The founder of the Ming dynasty had five poor Major Features, according to tradition. And some of the most famous people of today are similarly blessed. But keep in mind what the Chinese consider good:

· A long life with a happy old age
· Many children and grandchildren and great-grandchildren
· Money without having to work hard for it

Fame, success, power, excitement aren't in there.

As you learn about your own face, and what it represents, you have to consider what is good for you—for what you want out of life—and also how to work with your features and makeup to make the best impression on others to help realize your goals.

In the Chinese art of Face Reading you have five major elements to work with:

1. The Position Points—indicative of your present age and each with a special meaning in your destiny and personality.

2. The Palaces—each relates to a particular aspect of living.

3. The Three Stations—the top, middle and bottom sections of the face, representing respectively, youth, maturity, and old age.

4. The Five Major Features—the brows, the eyes, the nose, the ears, and the mouth—each revealing an aspect of your capacities.

5. The Seven Minor Features—the forehead, the undereye area, the cheekbones, the laugh lines, the groove from the nose to the upper lip, the jawline, and the chin—indicating your approaches to life challenges. Although called "minor," these features are very significant.

You will also consider the color of the various parts of the face: the hair—how it grows, its texture, thickness, and shine; facial lines—whether at the corners of your eyes, on your forehead, or around your mouth (many of these lines are assets); and above all, whether the face and features have balance and harmony.

To achieve harmony, consider your current Position Point and other elements one by one, but also view the face as a whole and understand how the features balance each other or cancel one another out.

Your Position Point

THE POSITION POINTS represent your current place in life (indicated by your age and its corresponding point) and also have special significance as to what life has to offer you—travel, children, a home, prosperity, success.

As we have noted, each of the numbered points—Position Points —represents a year in your life, beginning with the time of birth— Point 1.

To understand what your life is like at the present moment—or to understand the current state of anyone you are interested in and whose age you know—study the Position Point that represents your *current age plus one*.

The reason for *plus one* is that the Chinese assume that a person is one year old at the day of birth, for they add onto the life span the time that is spent in the womb. So our Western first birthday is Position Point 2; the year of our twentieth birthday is Position Point 21—and so on. The Chinese Position Point is always one year ahead of ours.

To find your current Position Point, add one year to your current age and see where this number appears on the Map of the Face. Keep this point in mind till your next birthday, when your Position Point advances by one.

WHAT DOES THE POSITION POINT SIGNIFY?

First, your current Position Point is an indication of present vitality. If you are healthy and in good emotional balance, your Position Point shows a pinkish glow. Keep an eye on it. If it becomes pale or grayish or greenish, your vitality may be diminishing—you may need more exercise, more fun, more relaxation. Although you may not at first be aware of anything perceptible about this point, as you pay it your attention, you (and others) will be able to discern any slight changes in its quality that will help you keep yourself in an optimum emotional and physical state. If you have a blemish or scar or mole at this point, it may indicate a year in which to watch out for hazards, or, depending on what the point signifies, other meaningful events in your life.

The Position Point also indicates where you now stand in your life pattern and what qualities you should be developing in yourself, and what areas you should emphasize or deal with in your career, makeup, and personality. It helps spell out your goals for this year in your life. As you will see, your Position Point should be considered in relation to which of the three Stations it falls and also to the meaning of the feature—mouth, forehead, eyes, nose, cheekbones—it may occupy. For example, any point on the forehead has to do with youth and your endowments; any point on the nose has to do with achievement in the middle years.

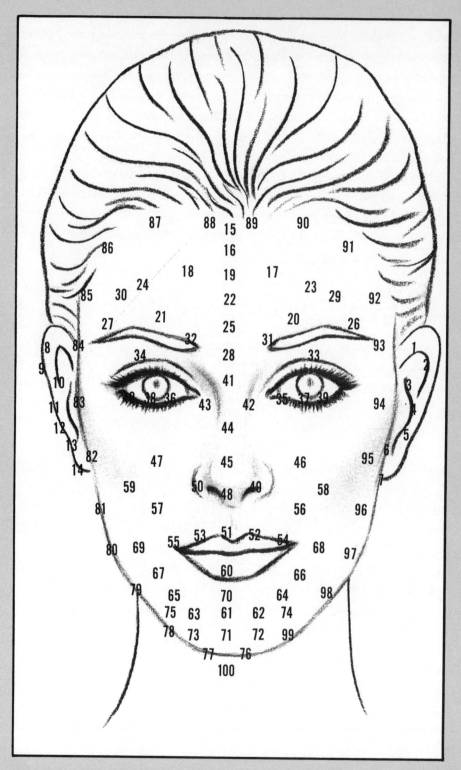

THE MAP OF
THE FACE. *Each
number—Position
Point—represents a
year in the life. Your
present Position
Point is your age on
your next birthday—
your current age
plus 1. The numbers
around the outside
of the face—76 to
100—also represent
the animal signs of
the Chinese zodiac.*

Position Points also have meanings of their own and provide check-points for various activities. Position Points 31 to 34 indicate chances for success in your career. The "stage coaches," the areas around Points 27 and 26, are travel signifiers, and their quality with that of point 61 should be checked if you are planning a trip. Points 68 and 69 are "society points." If one of these is emphasized, it indicates you are a good socializer and a favored conversationalist. Point 28, Shrine of the Seal of Heaven is an indicator of public acclaim.

Position Points 17 and 18 are respectively the "sun point" and the "moon point," and together are called "parent points"—the sun representing the father and the moon the mother. They indicate how you treat your parents, and this, as you know, tells a lot about how you deal with others in the world around you.

Point 44 is the "age point" and indicates the state of health; Point 45 is the "longevity point" and with other factors relates to the length of your life.

The face also has Star Points, which are not Position Points but areas surrounding certain Position Points. Star Points signify high-lights in one's life, so if your Position Point falls in one of these areas, it will signify an important period. (See the illustration on page 32.) The Star Points surround Points 25 and 28, between the brows; Point 41, the area between the eyes; the entire brow area (surrounding Points 31–33, 32–34); and the whole eyes (Points 35, 37, 39 and 36, 38, and 40). Glow and good color in these areas are a promise of good luck and good health; poor color (grayish, greenish, yellowish) should be considered a caution sign. This color does not, of course, refer to the color of the *iris,* the colored part of the eye.

You can also use your present Position Point as a personal focus. It is not necessary to call attention to it in any specific way. It is a good idea, though, to use it as your personal reference point, for whatever that may mean for you. In a way, it is your "home" for this particular year. Your next year will focus on another point—perhaps on the other side of your face, perhaps in a different Station or relating to a different feature, marking inward as well as outward change. One subtle way in which this change might work: When your Position Point is on your left side (Point 23, for example), resemblances to your father's side of the family and activities related to your father's influence may come out; when the Position Point advances to the right side (Point 24), your resemblances to your mother and your mother's influence may be stressed. When your Position Point reaches the middle of the face (Point 25), you feel more like your own person. If you are meditating with the object of achieving body harmony, you might focus upon your current Position Point as a unifying influence. This may help bring a glow to the point.

The Position Points as shown on the Map of the Face will also be used as reference points for applying cosmetics. For example, blusher should be placed so it goes no lower than Points 58 and 59 on the cheeks, and no nearer the nose than Points 46 and 47.

Primarily, the Position Points indicate what is happening in your current year. As you see, Position Points 1 to 7—representing birth and early childhood—appear on the left ear, and these indicate the influence of the father. Position Points 8 to 14—representing puberty —appear on the right ear and indicate the influence of the mother.

Position Points 15 to 33 (youth and young adulthood) appear on the forehead, representing your background and heredity.

Position Points 33 to 44 (early maturity) cluster around the brow and eye areas, and pertain to your reputation, intelligence, and inner energy.

Position Points 45 to 50 (the middle years) appear on nose and cheekbones—the areas of achievement.

Position Points 51 to 60 (maturity) surround the mouth (with the exceptions of Points 58–59, which are in the hollows of the cheeks) and indicate personality and productivity.

Position Points 61 to 75 (prime of life) are mostly on the chin, the area of strength.

Position Points 76 to 100 wrap around the outside of the face. These represent not only old age but the animal signs of the Chinese zodiac.

The Position Points with their names are listed here so you can understand the significance of your present year. Those with special significance are enlarged upon as we discuss the various features and stations they relate to.

THE 100 POSITION POINTS

Each Position Point has a particular significance to your destiny. Note the Star Point areas indicating your chance to "star"—and the Planet Points, representing a new phase, or passage, in your life.

1. Ear Points

The ears hold the age points of childhood. The left ear is the Wheel of Heaven and the right the Wheel of Humanity. Moving together, the two Wheels create life. The ears are Planet Points; the left ear representing Jupiter (wood); the right ear, Venus (gold). Here are points 1 through 14:

> 1, 2, Upper Wheel of Heaven
> 3, 4 Middle Wheel of Heaven
> 5, 6, 7 Heavenly Pearl Drop
> 8, 9 Upper Wheel of Humanity
> 10, 11 Middle Wheel of Humanity
> 12, 13, 14 Pearl Drop of Humanity

2. Forehead Points

The forehead holds the age points of youth and early adulthood— when you get your education, separate from your parents, travel, and establish your identity.

> 15 Mars (fire)—aggression, intensity, positive force (a Planet Point).
> 16 Middle Sky—a masculine, paternal point; finding of identity.
> 17 Sun Point—Father.
> 18 Moon Point—Mother.
> Together Points 17 and 18 are "parent points" and represent how you treat your parents.
> 19 Court of Heaven—maternal, feminine point; time of being "presented at court," making your entrance into society, acceptance as a grownup.
> 20, 21 Assistants, or Deputies—taking over responsibility from parents; a time when you assist others and learn from them

as a way of making your own place in the world.

22   Steward of Heaven—coming of age, maturity, taking your place in the world as a citizen.

23, 24   Lands That Lie to the Side (outskirts)—traveling, exploring, moving in and out of business and social environments, getting experience of the world.

25   Center of Heaven—the midpoint, where you assume control of your own destiny (a Star Point area).

26   Monument.

27   Mausoleum.

Points 26 and 27 are not "death" points. Rather they are "travel points," and are designated as they are, perhaps, because visiting the shrines of one's ancestors was a chief reason for traveling in ancient China.

28   Shrine of the Seal of Heaven—the most important point on the forehead, the point where you achieve fame, true adulthood, and self-responsibility, the "seal of approval" (a Star Point area).

29   Mountain or Highland—reaching a high point, experiencing the ups and downs of life; travel.

30   Forest—experiencing the wandering in and out, or searching, that one does after having reached a high point; travel.

3. Brow Points

These are points where you establish a family and your position in life. The brows (left and right) are Star Points.

31   Purple Air—honor and fame.

32   Floating Cloud—a time when you should be on "cloud nine."

33   Colorful Rainbow—the separating out of the essential parts of life, as light by a prism.

34   Kaleidoscope of Color—a colorful time of forming new patterns. Together Point 33 and 34 are called the *Rainbows*.

4. Eye Points

The eye points represent the two aspects of the Universal Energy— the creative or positive force, Yang (light), and the receptive Yin (dark). The left eye represents Yang and the right eye Yin. By analogy these points represent your inner force, vitality, or intelligence. Each entire eye is a Star Point: the left eye is Sun Star and the right eye is Moon Star.

35   Yang—positive early stage of development
36   Yin—receptive early stage of development
37   Middle Yang—positive middle stage of development
38   Middle Yin—receptive middle stage of development
39   Late Yang—positive third stage of development
40   Late Yin—receptive third stage of development

5. Nose and Cheek Points

These points represent accumulation of wealth and power.

41   Root of the Mountain—the beginning of life achievement, or success (A Star Point area, called Moon Dust)
42   Delicate Cottage—a place of seclusion and intimacy
43   Bright Palace—a place of much sociability and entertainment
44   Sitting on Top of One's Age—achieving control of one's health and position
45   Sitting on Top of One's Longevity—planning for the fruits of old age
46   East Mountain
47   West Mountain
     (Points 46 and 47, the cheekbones, represent power.)
48   The Peak of Perfection—the height of achievement (a Planet Point—Saturn, Earth)
49   Balcony—a place from which you look out upon the world
50   Pagoda—a landmark that is visible from a distance

6. The Philtrum Point

This point governs the groove from the nose to the upper lip and represents productivity and sexuality because it is the channel between the male (nose) and female (mouth).

51   Center of Life—productivity

7. Mouth and Cheek Points

Points 52 through 55 all represent storing up. This is a time in life when you accumulate resources and store up the results of your previous efforts. Points 56 through 59 represent adjustments; point 60 (the mouth) personality.

52 Warehouse—the place of possessions, things to be kept.

53 Storage Area—the place of merchandise, things to be disposed of.

54 Food Depot—place where food (the nutrients of life) is stored.

55 Strong Room—place where valuables are stored.

56, 57 Law and Order (the laugh lines)—placing your life in order, conforming to the rules, to have a long life before you.

58, 59 Tiger's Ears—so named because these cheek points become tufted sometimes in people at this age. If ever you are to be a tiger, you should be one now.

60 Mercury (water of life)—personality (a Planet Point).

8. Chin and Jaw Points

These points represent a time when you receive rewards and honors due you.

61 Sea of Wine—fullness, travel in comfort.

62, 63 Cellars, basements—what underlies the foundations of life.

64, 65 Pools of Water—calmness, serenity, time of contemplation.

66, 67 Golden Robes—receiving of honors (such as the gold watches received at retirement).

68, 69 Return—start of second childhood. What you put forth in your life comes back to you. These are "society points," indicating sociability.

70 Court of Justice—if you are ever to be wise and have good judgment, this is the time.

71 Buried Treasure—what you have gathered together of value.

72, 73 Servants, helpers—now you need to rely on others for

daily needs.

74, 75   The Jawbone—status in life; position achieved.

9. *The Points of the Perimeter*

Position Points 76 through 100, running around the outside of the face, represent not only a year in the life of those who live that long, but, more generally, the twelve Earthly Branches—the animal signs of the Chinese zodiac. Each sign embraces two points, and represents, as do Western zodiac signs, approximately one month on the calendar, and two hours of the day. If you know your Western zodiac sign, you can find the corresponding animal signifier of the Chinese zodiac, and discover what position points belong to your particular sign. If you know your *time* of birth, you can find the Chinese animal sign that rules your birth hour (corresponding to the rising sign in Western astrology). Also observe which of the Three Stations your birth sign (and rising sign) occupy. And, because each of the Chinese animal signs rules, in sequence, a year as well, repeating in twelve-year cycles, you may also want to know the animal symbol for the year you were born (see chart below). The time of day ruled by the position points for the sign of the year, month, and hour of your birth may prove fortuitous for your various enterprises.

Position Point	Animal Symbol	Corresponding to	Hour of day or night
76, 77 (100)	Rat	Aries	11 p.m.–1 a.m.
78, 79	Ox	Taurus	1 a.m.–3 a.m.
80, 81	Tiger	Gemini	3 a.m.–5 a.m.
82, 83	Hare	Cancer	5 a.m.–7 a.m.
84, 85	Dragon	Leo	7 a.m.–9 a.m.
86, 87	Snake	Virgo	9 a.m.–11 a.m.
88, 89	Horse	Libra	11 a.m.–1 p.m.
90, 91	Goat	Scorpio	1 p.m.–3 p.m.
92, 93	Monkey	Sagittarius	3 p.m.–5 p.m.
94, 95	Cock	Capricorn	5 p.m.–7 p.m.
96, 97	Dog	Aquarius	7 p.m.–9 p.m.
98, 99	Boar	Pisces	9 p.m.–11 p.m.

THE ANIMAL SYMBOL FOR THE YEAR OF YOUR BIRTH

The Animal Symbols for the years 1900 to 1995 are given here. If you were born between January 1 and February 19 of any year, note this important difference between the Western New Year and the Chinese New Year. The Chinese New Year does *not* start on January

Symbol	Year (with starting date of new year)			
Rat	1900 (1–31)	1912 (2–18)	1924 (2–5)	1936 (1–24)
Ox	1901 (2–19)	1913 (2–6)	1925 (1–25)	1937 (2–11)
Tiger	1902 (2–8)	1914 (1–26)	1926 (2–13)	1938 (1–31)
Rabbit	1903 (1–29)	1915 (2–14)	1927 (2–2)	1939 (2–19)
Dragon	1904 (2–16)	1916 (2–3)	1928 (1–23)	1940 (2–8)
Snake	1905 (2–4)	1917 (1–23)	1929 (2–10)	1941 (1–27)
Horse	1906 (1–25)	1918 (2–11)	1930 (1–30)	1942 (2–15)
Sheep	1907 (2–13)	1919 (2–1)	1931 (2–17)	1943 (2–5)
Monkey	1908 (2–2)	1920 (2–20)	1932 (2–6)	1944 (1–25)
Cock	1909 (1–22)	1921 (2–8)	1933 (1–26)	1945 (2–13)
Dog	1910 (2–10)	1922 (1–28)	1934 (2–14)	1946 (2–2)
Boar	1911 (1–30)	1923 (2–16)	1935 (2–4)	1947 (1–22)

Symbol	Year (with starting date of new year)			
Rat	1948 (2–10)	1960 (1–28)	1972 (2–15)	1988 (2–17)
Ox	1949 (1–29)	1961 (2–15)	1973 (2–3)	1989 (2–6)
Tiger	1950 (2–17)	1962 (2–5)	1974 (1–23)	1984 (2–2)
Rabbit	1951 (2–6)	1963 (1–25)	1975 (2–11)	1985 (2–20)
Dragon	1952 (1–27)	1964 (2–13)	1976 (1–31)	1986 (2–9)
Snake	1953 (2–14)	1965 (2–2)	1977 (2–18)	1987 (1–29)
Horse	1954 (2–3)	1966 (1–21)	1978 (2–7)	1990 (1–27)
Sheep	1955 (1–24)	1967 (2–9)	1979 (1–28)	1991 (2–15)
Monkey	1956 (2–12)	1968 (1–30)	1980 (2–16)	1992 (2–4)
Cock	1957 (1–31)	1969 (2–17)	1981 (2–5)	1993 (1–23)
Dog	1958 (2–18)	1970 (2–6)	1982 (1–25)	1994 (2–10)
Boar	1959 (2–8)	1971 (1–27)	1983 (2–13)	1995 (1–31)

1. Instead, the Chinese New Year begins on the date of the new moon in the Sign of the Dog (Aquarius)—and this date varies from year to year. If your birthday falls in January or early February, check the date bracketed *after* your birth year. If your birthday falls *before* this date, your Animal Symbol is that of the preceding year—you may be a Dragon, not a Snake; a Tiger, not a Rabbit. For example, a person born before February 18 of 1958 was born in the Year of the Monkey, not the Year of the Cock.

The Twelve Palaces—Indicators of Present Fortune

THE PALACES OF THE FACE are various areas you can check to discover the prospects of success in your current life and the favorable or not-so-favorable auspices under which you engage in various enterprises—travel, marriage, friendship, children, career, and so on. Although the Palaces sometimes include Position Points, the meaning of the Palace applies to your current ventures, regardless of your present age and where your current Position Point falls. However, if your present Position Point does fall within a particular Palace, the affairs of that Palace will be of special importance in your current life.

If you are interested in a certain venture or area of experience, check the particular Palace that governs such events. If the color of the skin in the Palace is good and the area is glowy, you can expect good fortune. If the color is poor (or wrong for the area), or if the Palace appears dark and sunken, or blemished, you are warned of disappointment and had best delay or change your plans.

1. Palace of Achievement

This occupies the middle of the forehead and runs from Position Point 15, the Point of Mars (fire) through Position Point 25, the Center of Heaven (Middle Sky), and includes Position Points 16, 19 (the

THE TWELVE PALACES. The
Twelve Palaces are checkpoints for the
auspices—fair or foul—for your current
undertakings. Glow in these areas and
appropriate color suggests success in
your efforts.

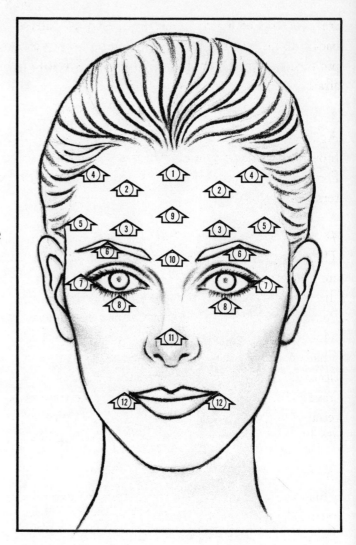

Court of Heaven) and 22 (the Steward of Heaven). As the forehead
is ruled by Mars, whose color is red, success is indicated when this Palace is pink and glowy.

2. Palace of Parents

There are two and they lie to both sides of the Palace of Achievement,
occupying the areas surrounding Points 17 and 20 on the left side
(father) and Points 18 and 21 on the right (mother). These Palaces

are indicators of matters relating directly to parents but also to your background, education and preparation for career. A pink glow is promising; too pale or too red, these areas warn of problems in such affairs.

3. Palace of Friends and Siblings

Again, there are two; they occupy the area above the inner part of the brow, surrounding Point 31 on the left, and Point 32 on the right. For success in matters concerning friendship and/or brothers and sisters, these areas should be pink and glowing.

4. The Palace of Transfer

There are two of these "transfer points" or "stage coaches" and they are indicators of travel, movement from place to place. They occupy the areas above the outer tip of the brows on both sides, including Points 26 and 27 (the Monument and Mausoleum), 29 and 30 (the Mountain and the Forest), and 23 and 24 (the Outskirts or Lands That Lie to the Side), and fill the entire triangle from above the brow tip to the hairline beyond the temple. Check these areas if you plan travel or anything involving movement or transfer of goods and materials. Prospects are good if these areas are pink and glowing; if they are discolored or greenish, your plans will not go well.

5. Palace of Happiness and Good Fortune

This covers the areas at the tip of the brow extending to the temple— surrounding Points 92 and 93 (the Monkey) on the left and Points 84 and 85 (the Dragon) on the right—and can be checked when you are involved in games of chance or other affairs dependent on luck, or whenever you face the prospect of happiness and good fortune.

6. Palace of Property

The areas governing property lie below the brow and include the Rainbow Points—33 and 34. Check these areas when you consider buying or selling, or if you are concerned with the value of property or are engaged in a career involving property. Those in the real estate business often have a very full, fleshy formation in these underbrow areas.

7. Palace of Marriage

Look for marriage prospects in the crow's-feet areas at the outer corners of the eyes. The corner of the left eye is the Palace of Wives and Children (marriage) and the corner of the right eye is the Palace of Concubines (extramarital affairs). The more crinkles you find here, the more marriages or extramarital affairs you can expect to indulge in. Smooth Palaces of Marriage give contentment.

8. Palace of Offspring

The areas underlying both eyes are the Palace of Children. This area is said to take a special glow when a woman is pregnant. Dark color indicates sexual overindulgence.

9. Palace of Life

This place of vitality lies between the brows, surrounding Point 28—the Shrine of the Seal of Heaven. This area is also a Star Point. A purplish glow in this area is said to denote fame and good fortune. Use it as a vitality checkpoint when energy is needed for an endeavor.

10. Palace of Health

This sits between the brows upon the Root of the Mountain (Point 41), and is the indicator of physical well-being. Check this area for any signs of physical disorder. For example, a line or dull color here can be the sign of fatigue or diminishing strength. Good color and smoothness signify health and free energy flow.

11. Palace of Wealth

The tip of the nose, including Point 45 (Longevity), Point 48 (the Peak of Perfection), and also the nostrils (Point 49, the Balcony, and Point 50, the Pagoda), is the Palace of Wealth. The "good" color for this area is golden peach—the color of Saturn (Earth). A full round well-built Palace of Wealth is promising for accumulation of money. Check this area for all money ventures, including expenditures. Too red, it can indicate impulsiveness, extravagance; greenish, money loss and financial woes.

12. Palace of the Household

This occupies most of the chin, including the Points 51 through 70. This area was originally called the Palace of Servants and Slaves, but of course people no longer have slaves and servants. It is actually the Palace of Management—governing the whole business of living. You would check this area for the state of your affairs; for indications of how your personal habits, relationships with those who work with you, who perform services for you, and for whom you perform services are affecting your well-being. Also for the management of your body, your mineral reserves, and physical functioning; and how this affects your strength and fortitude. Fullness and good firm flesh in this Palace indicate a well-functioning and well-managed life.

Star Points

THERE ARE SIX STAR POINTS. The area surrounding Position Point 28 is called Purple Air. (Do not confuse it with Position Point 31, also called Purple Air, which is adjacent to this Star Point.) A purplish glow here promises success, fame. Star Point 2 (Moon Dust), surrounds Position Point 41, and also augurs success, especially if there is *width* in this area. Each brow is a Star Point. The left brow is the Baron, or Overlord; the right brow is the Counselor. The brows are violent stars and should not be allowed to intrude into other Star Point areas. For this reason, keep adequate space between your brows to clear the Purple Air Star Point area. The left eye is Sun Star; the right eye, Moon Star. Brightness in these Star Points indicates intelligence, inner vitality.

It is of particular significance to your present life to know where your current Position Point falls, what Palace, Star Point, or Feature it is related to, in which of the Three Stations it lies, and which side of the face—left, father; right, mother—influences it. Or is it in the middle of the face, meaning a self-oriented year?

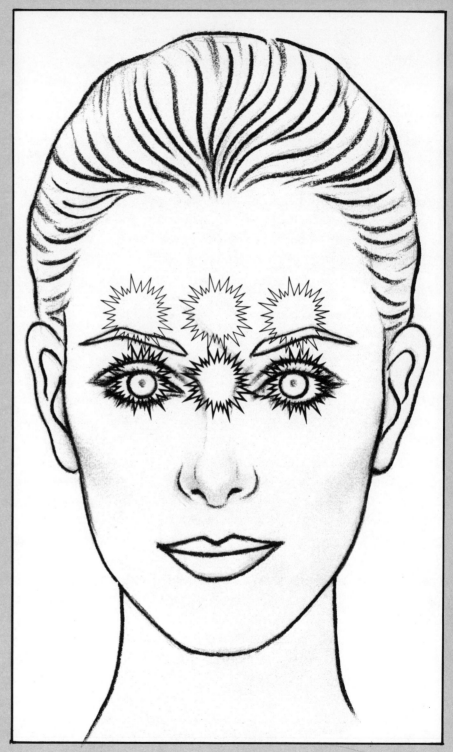

THE SIX STAR POINTS. The six Star Points are indicators of your chances to achieve success, fame. When your Position Point is on a Star Point, you can look for a change in your fortune—for better or for worse.

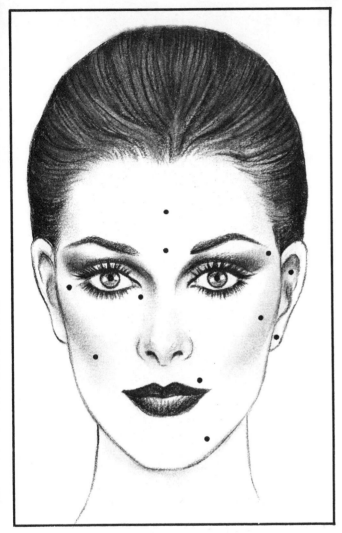

BEAUTY MARKS. Moles—beauty marks—have varying significance, depending on their location. Most moles on the face—exposed moles— are not considered lucky, but people with facial moles often have a corresponding hidden (fortunate) mole on the body.

MOLES

Moles have varied meanings, depending on where they are placed.

- A mole at Position Point 22 in the middle of the forehead indicates high achievement but someone who is too aggressive to stay married.

- Beside the eye, a mole is considered attractive, romantic, sexy, but its owner may be fickle in love, even adulterous.

- At Position Point 42 or 43, we find the weeping mole. The person with this mole tends to have health problems.

- A mole at Position Point 93 (or 84) at the outer tip of eyebrow indicates travel and movement in life.

- Ear moles are very good. Those at Points 3 or 7 or 10 or 14 tell of high achievement, a very fortunate life with money and good family.

- At Point 94 (or 83) just inside the cheek, a mole gives power and strength.

- Moles at Points 68 and 69, the "society points," show someone who is fortunate, sociable, but not always reliable.

- A mole at Point 28 (between the brows) is called "two dragons clasping the pearl." If it is a bright shiny mole (not a dullish one), it indicates a woman who can achieve high position, maturity, sophistication.

- Moles at Position Points 54 or 55 at the corner of the upper lip are "gourmet moles," indicating someone who enjoys food and the good things of life.

- Near Points 64 or 74 (or 65, 75), you find the "matchmaker's mole." This indicates a very colorful person, perhaps a busybody. In the theater, when this kind of character is played, a mole is placed here to indicate her role.

2. The Three Stations

IN CHINESE FACE READING the face is separated lengthwise into Three Stations:

- The First Station—the top of the face from hairline to midbrow—represents your background, mentality, and attitudes toward life and youth.

- The Second Station—the middle of the face, from the browline to the tip of the nose—represents adulthood, achievement, capacity, what you do for yourself with your life.

- The Third Station—the lower part of the face, from tip of nose to chin—represents maturity, what you have achieved, longevity, health, children.

When these Three Stations are in balance, the individual is said to be in harmony. When a hairdresser is working with your hair style to "make your face approximate the ideal oval," he or she is actually trying to make these Three Stations appear in harmony. When you have learned how to balance your face with hairdo and makeup, you present yourself to others as a more balanced, harmonious personality, and gather the benefits of more generous attitudes. Besides, by visualizing yourself as a balanced personality, you help free yourself from tensions and create greater harmony within yourself. You gain in confidence.

We'll go further into face balancing with hairdo and accessories in chapter 7. But an understanding of the meaning of the Three Stations and how they relate to your makeup and your fortune is needed to get you started.

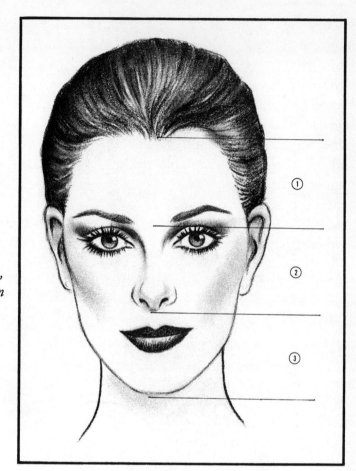

THE THREE STATIONS. Each Station represents a significant part of your life—Station 1, top of the face, youth; Station 2, middle face, the middle years; and Station 3, lower face, the later years. When the Stations are in balance, the life is in harmony.

STATION 1

Youth-oriented people have a dominant First Station. The First Station holds Position Points 15 through 32 and so represents the years of adolescence and young adulthood. Position Points 85 to 92 that run around the hairline represent the years in life that are often spent in recollection of youth—second childhood.

The First Station embraces only one Minor Feature—the forehead. But it holds some very important Position Points and Palaces. The most significant area of the First Station is formed by Position Points 15, 16, 19, 22, and 25—called the Palace of Achievement. The smoothness and good color of this area indicates an ability to succeed in official capacities. If you are to seek political work or a civil service job, Point 25 on your forehead should be glowy. Point 28 is the signifier of fame—the Shrine of the Seal of Heaven. If the area between your brows is wide and smooth and this area has prominence, it gives the ability to achieve social success and a high position. Career-minded women should pay particular attention to this Position Point and the whole Palace of Achievement. The Palaces of Parents, Siblings and Friendships and the Stage Coaches—Palaces of movement, travel—are also in this area.

A well-shaped, broad and high First Station gives the impression of intelligence, youth, and vitality that leads to success.

If you are between the ages of fourteen and thirty-two, the First Station is the significant one to your present life, and your current accomplishments depend on the qualities that it represents.

STATION 2

Success-oriented people have a dominant Middle Station. They are self-achievers. This Station occupies the space from the browline to the tip of the nose and represents adulthood, career, achievement— what you are capable of doing with your life. This Station is especially significant because it includes four Major Features (the eyes, the nose, brows, and even the ears) and two Minor Features (the cheekbones and undereye areas). The years of the thirties and forties that fall in this Station are the time of achievement and realization of life goals, whether in career or family life. Obviously, it is a period when emphasis in makeup should be upon the eyes. Point 41, the area between the eyes—the Root of the Mountain—is an indicator of health and also shows domestic harmony or disharmony. Position Points 41, 44, 45, and 48 on the nose concern success in work and accumulation of wealth. The Palaces of Health, Wealth, Happiness, Property, Marriage, Children fall in the Second Station.

If your current Position Point falls in the Second or middle Station, you should be concerning yourself with achievement in your work, whether it is as homemaker or in a career, or a combination of both.

STATION 3

The lower part of the face, from the tip of the nose to the chin, the Third Station, represents maturity, what you can expect to achieve, health, longevity, and children. Family-oriented people have a dominant Third Station. The Third Station includes one Major Feature—the mouth, representing personality—and four Minor Features—the groove (Position 51) from the nostrils to the upper lip, which represents productivity, children and sexuality; the chin, strength; the jawline, position in life; and the laugh lines, longevity. The quality of life in old age—indicated by fecundity and the number of children you have produced to take care of you—is shown by this Third Station. Interestingly, Position Points 51 to 55—a time when women as well as men often cut loose and seek a new love—are indicators of stored energy, sexual vitality, the number of children, and vitality in old age. The Palace of Household (security) occupies the middle part of this station.

As the Third Station has much to do with the quality of life—and also one's appearance and personality in the final third of life—it is important to think about it while you are still young. This includes caring for the teeth so that the mouth will hold its shape in later years; maintaining a good diet to preserve the bones of the chin and jaws; taking the responsibility that firms the chin and jaw; developing a cheerful disposition that strengthens the laugh lines (longevity). And of course, having children in youth so that you will have grandchildren to enjoy in later years is part of the promise of the Third Station. The Third Station is the slowest to mature and its shape is subject to change as you grow older.

If your present Position Point falls in the Third Station, you will be chiefly concerned with personality, health, status, and well-being.

To evaluate the Three Stations, look for the balance or disparity among them. Ideally, the Three Stations should be of equal length and of balanced width. This means that all three areas of your life will be productive and rewarding and will bring you happiness.

Not all of us of course have this ideal face. If the Stations are not exactly the same length—if one is more prominent, another smaller—it indicates the area in which you will have achievement or lack it.

- If the First Station (top of face) is long and the other Stations shorter, you will have a good beginning, but not do so well in the middle years or in old age.
- If the Second Station is short, you are perhaps not a self-achiever, and will rely on your family and others.
- If the Third Station is short, it is not favorable for a terrifically long
- life, and may bring problems in old age.
- If the Second Station is long but the First is relatively short, you may have a poor beginning, but find success in the middle years.
- If you have a strong Third Station, you will have a good long life with lots of children and a comfortable family situation. There are exceptions to this: too long a chin is not good—it can mean one is self-centered, and looks too much after oneself to achieve a reward-ing maturity.

You should also observe whether the Station is flat or rounded:

- If your First Station is flat rather than rounded, you will have to work hard to get started; if it is domed, or rounded, you will get more help from your family and background.
- If your Second Station is flat, you may never reach a position of power; a prominent nose and cheekbones help a rise in status.
- If your Third Station is flat, it may produce weakness in old age; a knobby chin and strong jaws contribute to longevity and strength.

The balance of the two sides of the face is also something to think about. Ideally, the two sides of the face should be the same size and shape, with no irregularities. Sometimes, though, there is weakness on one side or the other. As the left side represents the father, and the Yang or positive force in the universe, it demands strength for achieve-ment. The right side represents the mother, the Yin or receptive force in the universe, and requires yielding, a characteristic also necessary in getting along in the world. If either side is out of balance—stronger or weaker than the other—or if the nose or mouth or other Major Feature is crooked, your approach to life may be one of pushing too hard or yielding too much, whichever applies.

3. How to Find Your Face Shape

MANY WOMEN can't figure out their face shape. If you don't know your face shape, evaluating the Three Stations is the key. Look at your face straight on in a mirror and use a ruler if necessary to measure the three parts of the face. Another way is to hold a comb over one half of your face and see where you have width, narrowing and length.

- If the *Three Stations* are of about equal length, and equal width, somewhat narrower than they are long and the forehead hairline is somewhat squared off and the chin and jawline strong, you have an oblong face. The Chinese art of Face Reading considers this the "ideal" face because it gives equal value to the three periods of life —youth, maturity and old age. It means a long good life, with excess in nothing—the Chinese ideal of balance and harmony.

- If your *First Station* (top of the face) is wider than the other two Stations and your Third Station (bottom of the face) is narrower than the other two, you have a triangular face. This kind of face emphasizes youth—the need for achievement before age thirty. But it also indicates creativity, mental quickness, and perhaps a tendency to get lost in fantasy and to fail to put dreams into reality.

- If your *Second Station* (midpart of the face) is wider than the other two Stations, and your Third Station is narrower than the First Station (top of face), with the chin pointed and the hair growing into a peak on the forehead (considered lucky!), you have a heart-shaped face. The first half of your life will be the stronger and you should try to establish yourself before you are forty. However, because of your width at the cheekbones, you usually have more vital-

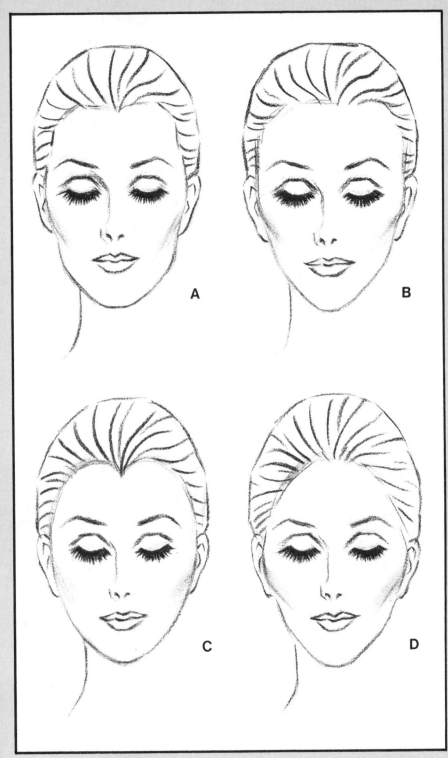

(A) OBLONG FACE. Each Station is about the same length and width. This promises a balanced personality.

(B) TRIANGULAR FACE. The First Station is wide—often high—tapering to a small chin. This indicates creativity, mental alertness.

(C) HEART-SHAPED FACE. Wide middle Station, forehead peak, narrow chin. Gives charm, social grace.

(D) DIAMOND-SHAPED FACE. Wide cheekbones, narrow forehead, narrow chin. An achiever with success in middle years.

ity after thirty than the person with a triangular face. With this face you seek personal power, but oftener in the emotional areas of life rather than in public position.

· If your face is widest at the Second (middle) Station, and the forehead narrows toward the top midpoint and the chin is pointed, but the Three Stations are of about equal length, you have a diamond-shaped face. A diamond-shaped face is basically the same as heart shape, the only difference is that a diamond-shaped face usually belongs to a person with more prominent bone structure and without a widow's peak. Usually this face has a rounded forehead and high cheekbones. You are likely to find your greatest success in the middle years, but have little help from your family and background. In later years, your fortunes may decline (pointed chin).

· If your Three Stations are of about the same length and width—equally long and wide—and your hairline and jawline are squared off, you have a square face. This shows much persistency and achievement but you are a doer rather than a thinker and often self-centered.

· If your Three Stations are the same length and width, with the forehead and chin rounded off, you have a round face. This means you are easygoing, good tempered, and take things as they come without striving too hard for success.

· If your Third Station is wider than the other two Stations, and the Second and First Stations are of about equal length and breadth, you have a pear-shaped face. You may have to struggle in your early and middle years, but your third part of life will be productive, though you will probably try to dominate others.

· If the Second Station is wider than the other two Stations, with the Third Station somewhat narrower than the forehead and the chin rounded but small, you have an oval face. This is considered the ideal face for beauty. But because the chin is weak, the third part of life will not be rewarding. You should start thinking early of providing for your later years—because you learn to enjoy success and luxury while young. Many beauties with oval faces marry wealthy older men whose estates will provide for their future.

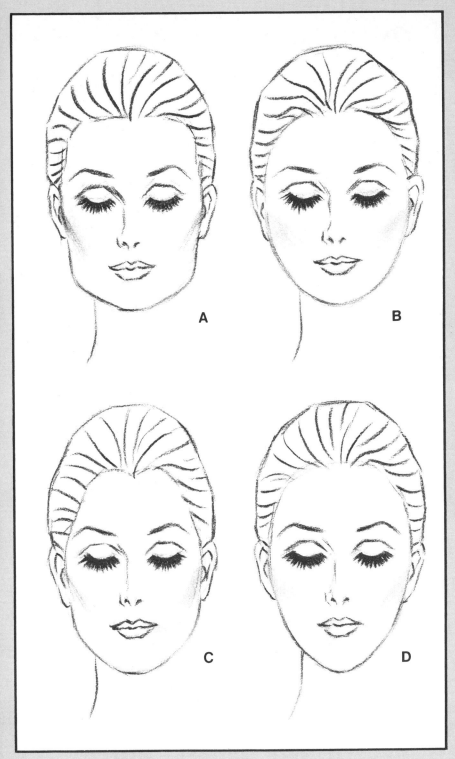

(A) SQUARE FACE. The Three Stations are about the same length and width and squared off. You are persistent—a doer, perhaps self-centered.

(B) ROUND FACE. The Three Stations are about the same length and width, but rounded. Easy-going, good-tempered.

(C) PEAR-SHAPED FACE. Wide jaw-bones, with the Third Station (lower face) dominant. Tendency to dominate others; success in later years.

(D) OVAL FACE. The Three Stations are the same length, but cheekbones slightly wider, forehead rounded, small chin. Ideal for beauty, but its promise may falter.

4. Complexion Color—Look Healthy, Look Happy

A HEALTHY, HAPPY-LOOKING FACE has various shades of coloring that are appropriate to the various areas. By subtly toning these areas, you can bring an overall harmony to your face. But with any adjustment in color and shape of a feature, it is a good idea to do the least possible to get your effect. The exceptions are the eyes, brows and mouth—for which you can do a lot.

Certain areas of the face represent the various planets and have a distinctive color that enhances them:

- The forehead, representing Mars, should be pinkish.

- The nose, representing Saturn, should be golden peach.

- The mouth, representing Mercury, should be rosy but not too red.

- The left ear represents Jupiter; the right ear, Venus. The ears should be pinky white, lighter than the face.

- The eyes represent the light of Heaven—the left eye, the sun; the right eye, the moon. The eyes should be brilliant and clear.

The thing to avoid in your choice of facial makeup is colors that are yellowish, greenish, grayish, brownish, dark. When any part of the face takes on these colors—notably the undereye area, but sometimes other areas—or if the nose or ears are too red, it is considered a sign either of disturbed metabolism or of emotional upset, and bodes ill for the area of the life covered by the Palaces or Position Points that are off-color.

BASIC MAKEUP

Before you choose a foundation, determine whether your skin is oily, combination oily and dry, or dry.

- If the skin is oily, choose a moisturizer that is water-based and a liquid foundation that is water-based.

- If skin is combination—oily in the "T" zone in the middle of the face, and dry elsewhere—still use a water-based moisturizer and foundation, but in the undereye area use an oil-base moisturizer.

- For a dry skin, use oil-base moisturizer and liquid foundation. Color selection is the same, no matter what your skin type.

- Test for foundation color on the skin of the inside of the wrist, where the skin color is closest to your basic skin tone. Avoid foundation that is too pink or too white. A beige or medium beige is usually best. Even if your skin is ruddy, don't choose a rose tone because you will only add more pink. You hardly ever go wrong if you choose a neutral color—neither too white nor too pink.

- Very young teenagers who are just starting to use makeup should not use a liquid foundation. Choose a water-base moisturizer and more transparent makeup—lip gloss and a transparent cream blush.

APPLICATION

Apply moisturizer first by the five-dot method—put a dot of moisturizer on Position Points 22 (forehead), 45 or 48 (on the nose), 46 and 47 (on the cheeks), and 71 (on the chin). Then gently blend with the fingertips so moisturizer covers the face completely. Now the skin is ready for makeup.

Dot the same five points with liquid foundation and again gently blend in with your fingertips. If any area needs more coverage—the undereye or the laugh lines and midforehead (Points 25 and 28) and usually around the nostrils (49 and 50) and middle of the chin (71,

76, and 77)—because the coloring is somewhat uneven there or there may be little lines, add a little coverup cream in addition to the liquid foundation.

Coverup cream should not be very white—if it is too light, it gives an owlish look to the eyes. Choose it in a medium to tan shade. It is intended to reflect light, not create a patchy area.

Once that is done, the face should look very even.

Now puff on a light loose powder to set the makeup so it won't streak. And do not be afraid of using a loose powder, because it does *not* go into the pores and will *not* dry your skin. It not only helps keep your makeup on all day, but also helps keep the natural moisture in, and if you use loose powder to set your foundation, your skin will not dry out as easily.

When that is done, your face is like a canvas, you are ready to go on to your pretty colors—brows, eyes, cheeks, lips.

Blusher should be rosy, pink, peach, tawny, or bronze, to go with your clothes color.

Eye colors and lip colors are fashion colors—they should be harmonized with your clothes. New shades of eye and lip makeup that come out seasonally are designed to harmonize with the fashion colors being promoted then and you need new eyeshadow and lipstick shades to keep your face in harmony with your wardrobe.

5. Emphasize the Positive— The Five Major Features

I**N BALANCING THE FACE,** you work with the Five Major Features and Seven Minor Features as well as with the Three Stations. The Five Major Features are:

- The brows—representing fame

- The eyes—representing intelligence

- The nose—representing wealth and opportunity

- The mouth—representing personality

- The ears—representing potential force and longevity

These features are "major" because they are the most prominent but also because, in Face Reading, they represent what you make of your own life. The art of Chinese Face Reading says that one good feature gives you ten happy years. In working with a woman's face, a makeup artist or a hairdresser always looks first for her best feature and builds a look around it. You can do this for yourself.

Every person has one very special feature. By recognizing this feature and understanding what it represents in your life, you work with your makeup to bring out the qualities of your personality that this feature points up and give yourself the benefit of your latent capacities.

You will also be calling the attention of others to your better qualities and tempting them to ignore the less favorable qualities that are also revealed in your face. At the same time, you draw the power of your own positive thinking to your assets rather than to your liabilities, both in appearance and the way you present yourself. This knowledge of the meaning of features is helpful, too, in evaluating the people you encounter, letting you better judge those you get to know socially, are attracted to or tend to avoid; it helps you understand those you work with, so you can get along better and know whom to trust.

The Eyebrows—Fame

THE EYEBROWS—the entire brow area—represent your reputation, your place in society, your claim to fame, your emotions, creativity, and achievement. They also reflect your relationship to those close to you; and perhaps more than any other feature, the eyebrows set the *mood* of your face. Luckily, they are the feature that is easiest to change—to reinterpret. You can lighten them or darken them; you can adjust their shape, thin them or make them heavier; lengthen them, shorten them. But unfortunately, they are also the feature that demands the most art in designing the line that is exactly right for your face. Fashions in eyebrows also change from time to time from dark to light, from heavy to thin. However, on the positive side, there are certain definite rules about brow shaping that you can follow— and you'll never go very wrong if you follow the rules given here for the ideal brow.

But first, let's look at *your* brows and see what you have to work with. It's a good idea to evaluate your brows as they look on your "naked" face—clean, no makeup, with your hair pulled back to expose your forehead and cheekbones. As a Major Feature, the brows help balance the rest of the face and should be in harmony with the strength and weakness of the other Major Features.

· The first thing you should make sure of is that the eyebrows don't run together right across the bridge of your nose. Although this might give strength and character to a male face, it is not considered lucky even for a man and is much too "hairy" for any standard of female beauty. As we have seen, the brows represent stars—but violent stars—and mustn't be allowed to invade other star territory.

- The second point is that the brows should have smoothness and line without straggly hairs above or below the natural arch.

- The brows should not be so bold that they dominate the face. They should be smooth, elegant and well-groomed.

So consider your natural brows in terms of how they reveal your own idea of beauty and the mood of your face. Do they make you look important, likely to dominate others by their strength? Or are they sparse and pale and show you to be someone who is likely to be shy and reclusive, to work behind the scenes and to let others push you around—maybe too much?

Neither extreme is ideal. But the brows frame the eyes and show how you relate to people, so work first with the basic shape of the brows and leave their thickness and color till you decide how much strengthening or subduing they need in order to balance your face and make a pleasing impression. Start by measuring your brows to find the ideal shape.

THE IDEAL BROW

The eyebrow is the frame for the eye—and ideally is long and elegant, smooth and delicately arched. It is slightly wider at the inner tip but preferably almost all the same width or thickness between the inner tip (nearest to the brow) and the height of the arch, and tapering only slightly to the natural end of the brow.

The brow follows the natural form of the brow bone that underlies it and it is best to work with this natural structure. If you follow your own natural brow bone, you can have the ideal brow for your particular face.

HOW TO SHAPE YOUR BROWS

Hold a pencil or makeup brush vertically over your face from the outer tip of the nostril to intersect the eyebrow. With a brow pencil, make a dot at the point where the brow is intersected. This is the inner point where the brow should begin. Repeat on other eye. Then tweeze all hairs between these two points.

Next hold a pencil vertically over the face so that the pencil passes the outer edge of the iris (the colored part of the eye) when you look straight ahead. Where the pencil intersects the brow, put another dot. This should be the highest point of the arch. This means that the top line of the brow should run from the starting point to its highest point at the pencil mark. Brush your brows so that you see this line clearly. Be careful of tweezing any hairs in the upper part of the brow as it may ruin the arch. Usually tweeze only the lower part of the brow. Below the bottom line of the brow, tweeze hairs as necessary to clean away stragglers and to equalize the thickness of the brow so that it rises to the point of the arch.

Now place a pencil across the face from the outer corner of the nose to pass over the outer tip of the eye and to intersect the tail of the brow. Put a pencil dot there. The brow tip should come no lower than this point. Brow hairs beyond this point should be tweezed. Also stragglers above the top line of the brows—again, be careful with the upper hairs—and below so that the tip of the brow tapers gently (do not thin it to a fine line).

Place the pencil across the brow—the inner and outer brow tips should be on approximately the same level. (This is for the *ideal* brow.)

Work on one eye at a time so that you have the ideal shape on one before you start the other. This gives you a chance to see the difference shaping the brow correctly can make.

If your brows are heavy, thin them from below the brow line to a more or less even width all the way along between the inner tip and the arch. Avoid too much heaviness at the inner tip of the brow, and do not make the outer part too thin. The arch should be marked but not too pronounced—often tweezing only a hair or two from below will emphasize the arch sufficiently.

Avoid eyebrows that are tweezed to a fine line, and *never* shave off your eyebrows and redraw them (as some inexperienced people have done). Too thin brows give a vapid, empty look that is inappropriate for women today.

Once you have found the ideal shape for your brows, keep them groomed by tweezing straggling hairs and brushing them straight up and then outward to smooth them into the natural line of the brow before applying makeup.

Note that the space between the brows should be fairly wide—about two fingers width unless eyes are very close together; then one-and-a-half fingers. This opens up the face and also clears the area between the brows. As this is the Star Point representing fame, you want it to be clear and "dazzling." In addition, the more space between the eye and the brow, the larger and more open the eye appears. The heavier the brow the more it takes the emphasis away from the eye itself. However, the brow should not be too insignificant when compared to the size of the nose and width of the cheekbones and jaw. Proportion and balance must be kept in mind.

When balancing your brows to your face, observe the brows of others that are in the public eye. Some notable examples of brows and their

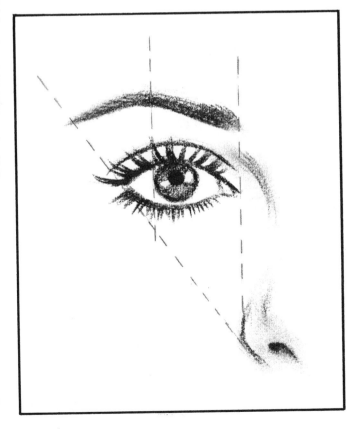

How to shape your brows: The inner tip of the brow should be directly above the outer edge of the nostril. The highest point of the arch, directly above the outer edge of the iris. The outer brow tip lies on a diagonal that passes from the outer edge of the nostril past the outer tip of the eye and intersects the brow.

relation to fame are these: Joan Crawford, whose pictures can still be seen on late-night movies, had very prominent brows in a time (the 1930s) when others (Garbo, for example) had pencil-line brows. Crawford's large, full eyes could carry the prominent brows that became her trademark. Crawford certainly rose from ignominy to fame, and as recent books about her indicate, dominated those around her; and after her acting days were done, she became a prominent executive for a major company. Garbo's high curved brow bone and delicate brows show her mysterious nature.

Today many models and actresses use their prominent brows as a trademark.

When you shape your own brows, consider your goals in life as well as the balance of your features. And also consider the impression that you will be making on others with your brows:

- The heavier and darker your brows, the more domineering but also effectual you will seem.

- The thinner and lighter your brows, the more adaptable and biddable but also less important you will appear.

- Long hairs within the brow after age forty show a long life. However, light shaggy brows with unruly hairs that stick out are considered a sign of sexual promiscuity. Any stubborn unruly hairs that stick out in a feminine brow should be tweezed. Your sexuality can be shown in other ways. This is, however, a sign to observe in a male partner; if you find it, expect only a light love; the owner of such brows is likely to be promiscuous. If, on the contrary, brows are smooth (and other characteristics indicate it), you can expect sexual fidelity.

- If hairs of the brow tip point upward, it indicates help from friends.

- Well-shaped smooth brows will make you appear confident and amenable, well groomed and intelligent, with emotions in control, and indicate a pleasant partner in life and love.

YOUR BROWS—THEIR MEANING AND MAKEUP

Your brows indicate your emotions, creativity, and achievement—your chance to achieve fame. Notice that Position Points 31, 32 (Purple Air, Floating Cloud) and 33, 34 (the Rainbows) are in the eyebrow area. This represents the time of life—early thirties—when one's position in life begins to become clear. It's the time when a person comes out into the public eye—the beginning of the middle, achievement period of life. It's therefore not so strange that women in their early thirties often "fix" their eyebrows for life, while younger women often don't do enough with their brows. Yet you should try to get your brows into ideal (for you) shape in the late teens and twenties, and those over thirty should realize that fashions in eyebrows change. Even though you have their basically ideal shape, you may need to modify it toward heaviness or thinness, darkness or lightness as the fashion of the time calls for. Today's fashion, for example, requires very little color to be added to brows.

BASIC BROW SHAPES

There are seven basic brow shapes, and an ideal formation for each type—and these brow shapes indicate the nature of the owner and her possibility for achievement in life. If you have definite life goals, you can adjust your brow shape to express them better. But this should be done within the basic natural framework of the brow. Often very minor changes get the result you want.

1. Arched Brow

This is the brow of beauty. You are born to the good things of life and can often acquire them with little effort. A brow with a pleasing natural arch indicates an artistic, romantic, and sensuous nature, but also a person of good character who will be successful in life. Once you have clarified its basic shape by measuring its ideal length and tweezing between the brows and at the tip and shaping up the arch, and tapering the outer tip, there is little you need to do to it. If the brow color is very light, you may want to darken it slightly. But still use a light brown pencil (be sure there is no reddish color in the pencil

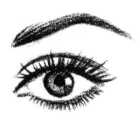

THE ARCHED BROW. Tweeze straggling hairs to clarify its basic shape. Indicates harmony in relationships.

unless the hair too has reddish tones). The arched brow is considered the ideal brow and indicates harmony in relationships.

2. *Upswept Brow*

This is the brow of the activist. The tail of this brow flies up into space, and it denotes one who is aggressive, sexy, enterprising, proud, and assured; but someone, too, who can be very determined in pursuit of a goal. Actually, this is a positive, optimistic brow and it may be not at all wrong if it is cleared and brought into a clean outline—though the outer tips of the brow will be higher than the level of the ideal brow. Sometimes, though, this brow may appear *too* aggressive. Then you can tweeze some hairs from the top of the outer tip and draw it down slightly. This brow can look threatening if it is too dark and heavy and if the inner tip comes down too close to the inner tip of the eye. Keep as much distance between the inner tip of the brow and the tip of the eye as you can. Tweeze a few hairs below the arch to indicate the arch more clearly and possibly draw in a few hairs above to give the upper brow line contour. Use a warm-tone highlighter on the brow bone below the outer tip. Take care, too, if you have this kind of brow, not to form the frown habit, drawing the inner tips of the brows together. If this brow is open and free, it can give you confidence and others will respect you as an achiever.

3. *Downswept Brow*

This is the brow of life's natural "victim." It is sometimes called the "wistful brow," because its owner seems to be begging for help. It is definitely not the sign of a doer and you must guard against a tendency to use sex—or helplessness—to achieve your goals. The problem with this brow is that others may think you are weak in character, dependent, selfish, even as they succumb to your seductions. If you want to get others on your side by pleading weakness rather than by showing strength, this eyebrow is helpful, for many people like to feel needed and others will pursue you, considering you must be sexually submissive. If it gets you into more bad situations than you like, you can modify it. Keep the outer tip thin and short (be sure it falls no lower than the mark of the pencil point on the brow-shaping diagram on page 51) and tweeze hairs below the natural arch to define

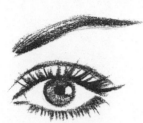
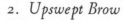

THE UPSWEPT BROW. *A positive, optimistic brow that may need only to be cleared and brought into a clean outline. The sign of an activist.*

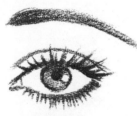
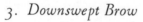

THE DOWN-SWEPT BROW. *Seductive. The outer tip needs to be thin and short. Place highlighter on the brow bone below the outer brow tip.*

an arch, filling in slightly above. Brush brow hairs of the tips up and out to give a more uplifted effect. Use a lighter highlighter on the brow bone beneath the outer brow tip. This bow is often seductive and pretty on the young, but may pull the whole eye area down with an aging effect as one gets older.

4. Short Brow

This is the brow of the ardent lover. With this brow, you are said to be passionate. Your strong points are ambition and independence. Your problems? Others may find you fickle and you tend to be short tempered. In appearance, this brow has a young look—and you may want to leave it that way if you are youthful enough to carry it off as an asset. Most people consider the youthful outlook of this brow to be attractive. In some faces, though, it seems only to bring out immaturity in character. If you want to change it, fill in the outer tip so that it tapers to the proper length (but do not bring it down too far or make it too heavy). Tweeze a hair or two below the natural high point of the brow to emphasize the arch and fill in slightly above the high point of the arch for a more sophisticated effect. This brow should be a nice medium thickness—too thin, it can become clownish; too thick, it can speak too strongly of the bluntness that tends to go with it. But you do accept challenges, and can achieve success.

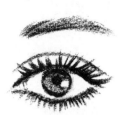

SHORT BROW.
This brow has a young look—and can be an asset. Keep it at a nice medium thickness—not too thick or too thin. This brow shows ambition, independence.

5. Level Brow

This straight brow is the brow of the career woman. You are impulsive, courageous, enjoy sports and the outdoor life, and are good at them and at your career. Unfortunately, you may be totally unfit for the traditional role of homemaker. This brow is common in the young because they are physically strong. Children have straight brows—and the brow tends to arch more as you grow older. Many young models have this brow. This is, however, the brow for a woman who wants to be challenged in her work, will be an outstanding executive and will meet men on their own level. Others are likely to accept you as being intelligent and competent—level headed. But they are likely to overlook your feminine needs, which you have, even if you aren't a cooky-baking mother. In fact, your nature makes you a perfect partner in a two-income household where both parents share the work

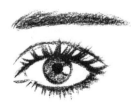

LEVEL BROW.
Soften a straight brow by keeping it light—or draw down a hair or two at the outer tip. This brow marks a career woman.

within and out of the home, because you're an organizer and can get things done efficiently and also are energetic.

If you want to modify your brows, draw a hair or two above the place of the natural arch (see diagram, page 51) and tweeze a hair or two below to create a contour. If the tip of the brow is high, you can draw down a hair or two at the outer tip. Another way to soften straight brows is to avoid darkening them—or even to lighten them if they are already dark. Try also to form the habit of raising your brows when you are concentrating instead of lowering them. It will make you appear more innocent and interesting, but not less efficient. Widen your eyes, too. Straight low brows sometimes appear scheming —which you really aren't. You simply plan the future with a clear vision.

6. Angular Brow

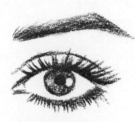

ANGULAR BROW. To modify the arch, tweeze one or two hairs above; fill in a little below the arch; keep the outer tip thin and tapering. Indicates a dramatic personality.

This wedge-shape brow is the brow of the adventurer. It shows you to be creative, brilliant in financial matters, with a long life ahead to achieve your goals. It is, let's face it, a buccaneering brow—and you tend to slash through obstacles to get what you want—and also to dominate any situation or relationship you're in. Because your needs in life are so various, you tend to be promiscuous—at least to need an occasional change of partner—and this won't make others happy. Weak men tend to lean on you, and unless you can use them for some immediate purpose, you are likely to ride roughshod over them. Strong men may try to break you, because you present a challenge. Anyway, your life is exciting and you are oriented to success. You have to realize that you are not always going to be trusted, and many women will consider you a rival, while men you meet in your career may feel threatened by you and regard you as dangerous and too strong competition. The wedge-shape brow certainly is *dramatic,* and you may want to emphasize it if you are in a cutthroat business— fashion, theater, and the like. Otherwise, you may want to soften it if it is too heavy, especially for the emotional part of your life.

Modify the arch by tweezing a few hairs above the arch to soften the sharp angle. Fill in slightly below the arch if needed by drawing in a few hairs and also soften the extension of the outer tip, by keeping it thin and tapering. Again, with the wedge-shape brow it is important to avoid the frown habit, because drawing your brows together can have a frightening effect. Softened and silky, these brows can be extremely beautiful and attractive—they make for an interesting face, no matter what else you've got or haven't got. Many women prefer to exaggerate such brows, rather than soften them; however, you do so at your own risk.

7. Rounded Brow

This is the brow of the businesswoman—the "operator." A woman with this kind of brow will be a canny business woman and perhaps an entertainer. The brows are almost perfect semicircles and rise above, usually, a nice fatty curve of the flesh over the brow bone. "Curved is the line of beauty"—so many people may think you are a self-indulgent and pampered person. In truth, you're resourceful, self-confident, and financially a wizard. You can make money on the stock market, in real estate, in buying and selling and at the bargaining table, or whatever. You always get away with the better part. You are also likely to be the dominant partner in a personal relationship, and are very shrewd as a judge of people and their motives. The important thing with this brow is not to thin it too much or it will look artificial.

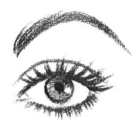

ROUNDED BROW.
A warm-tone high-lighter on the fatty part above the brow bone will soften the high arch of this "businesswoman" eyebrow.

Follow the shaping rules for the ideal brow, even if modifications here can be slight. Be sure neither tip comes too far down. Shape the curve to an almost straight line from the inner tip to the natural arch by drawing in a few hairs at the under side of the brow and flatten rather than raise the top of the arch; keep a straight line down at the brow tail or brush the hairs of the outer tip slightly out to reduce the down curve. A warm-tone highlighter on the fatty part above the brow bone will soften the high arch. Avoid extremes with this brow, so that it is neither too thin nor too thick, neither too dark nor too light, and note that what is usually done wrong with this brow is making it too curved and too thin. Because with this brow you will have a good eye for business, it is important to help others trust you. You'll probably marry for advantage and your mate will always do whatever you want him to do because you know exactly how to get around him. These are brows that tend to mesmerize because they combine astuteness with a seeming naïvete. You know what you want and the simplest way to get it. Usually what you want is money— and it is through sound business and possessions that you achieve prominence.

THE FINE ART OF BROW MAKEUP

Because your brows are so important to your beauty and to the impression you make on others, you should have the finest possible tools to shape them. These include:

· An eyebrow tweezer—one with a flat tip makes it easier to grasp the hair. The tweezer must have spring in the handle so it will hold the hair tightly when you remove it.

· Brow pencils in one or two colors. The pencil should be sharp, but not too sharp or it might redden the skin. If it's an automatic be sure it is well sharpened; if it is a wood-cased pencil, sharpen it flat to a razor-fine wedge edge.

· A stiff brow brush for grooming the brows.

How to Use a Tweezer

Once you have determined the basic points where your brows begin and end and the high point of the arch, you should tweeze the hairs that extend beyond these points at the inner and outer tip, and below the arch of the brow to get the desired shape. Before you start to tweeze, brush all the hairs of the brows up and then brush outward so they lie smoothly in the ideal shape of the brow.

· You need good light—and a firm rest for your elbow and a mirror that lets you get close to your eye, or else one that magnifies. Rest your elbow on the table and grasp one hair at a time in the tweezer and pull out in the direction that the hair grows. Be gentle but firm.

· Work from one eye to the other to be sure the shape is balanced on both eyes. Before you remove a hair, lift it up from the browline to be sure that removing it will not leave a "hole" in the brow.

· Work from the inner tip of the brow out and tweeze hairs only from below the line of the arch, tweezing as few hairs as possible to get the shape that you want.

· Use a little alcohol or witch hazel on the brow skin before you start to work to numb the slight pain you may feel from tweezing, and to reduce redness after tweezing.

If the skin becomes red and irritated after tweezing brows, tweeze at bedtime and after a hot bath or shower when the brow hair is softened by water and the pores are extended by heat.

Electrolysis is another means of removing brow hairs you know you want to be rid of forever. This is for hairs between the brows and stragglers above and below the arch and possibly for brow-tip hairs. Do not shape the entire brow permanently because styles in brows change and you may at some time want brows that are heavier than you now have and could have if tweezed hairs continue to grow in.

Penciling the Brows

Your brow pencil should be a light color. You use it to fill in the brow and point up its shape. It is not usually necessary to darken the brows unless they are very light blonde or white. Still, even in these cases use a shade of light beige or gray. The brow pencil should be *lighter* than your hair color.

· If you have light hair, use a gray or light brown pencil.

· If hair is medium dark, a light brown.

· If hair is very dark, you might use a dark brown or dark gray.

· Use a light black (charcoal) only if you have black hair and very dark skin.

· If hair is red or auburn, you can still usually use a light brown pencil as these colors often have a slightly warm reddish note.

· Use the pencil to fill in with a few light hairlike strokes where the brows are too thin and to extend them at the outer tip, possibly to raise the arch slightly. Use tiny hairlike upward strokes, and as few strokes as possible; never draw a hard line. Eyebrows are extremely delicate in their nuances and should always be handled with a delicate touch.

· Know when to stop. Less is better. Blend the filled-in areas with a brush for a still more natural look.

· Again, groom your brows by brushing them up and then brushing them outward into the line of your brows.

Once you have achieved the line of the brows that is right for you, leave them alone. Don't keep reshaping them. Of course, you will have to retweeze hairs as they grow in to maintain the line of the brow and to keep the brows neat, and from time to time as fashion changes in makeup or in your way of life, you require a new brow style. Just bear in mind you can easily be led into tweezing too much, making your brows too thin or creating holes in them. If you follow the basic plan for the length of your brows and point of the arch, and keep the brows proportionate to the other features of your face, you can have confidence in them—and others will have confidence in you.

Special Brow Problems

There are two other things that you can do with brows if you have special problems. You can lighten them. You can thin them.

If your brows are very dark and heavy and your skin is light and if you have lightened your hair extremely (or nature has), you may want to have your brows lightened. This can be done in a beauty salon or there are special eyebrow bleaches for home use. Lightening is often quite effective as it softens the brow hairs as well as softening the effect.

You can also have your brows dyed if they are too pale or if they are out of harmony with your hair color. It used to be the fashion (and may be again) to have brows dyed red if you colored your hair red, but this is no longer a fad. WARNING: Don't use hair dyes on your brows. Special brow dyes are available. Better, have the job done by a professional in a salon. Because brows grow at a slower pace than hair, the dyeing need be done only at intervals of several months.

Brows can also be thinned. If brow hairs are very bristly or contrary or grow in irregularly, and if from time to time heavy stray hairs appear along the brow line, they can be tweezed and the whole brow if necessary thinned. If this is done, the finer remaining brow hairs may be all brushed upward to define the arch without creating a heavy line. Many black women whose brow hairs may be very curly find this a good way to deal with the problem. But for many other women it also works well. It's a problem, though, to discuss with a beauty professional—unless you know exactly what you are doing.

It is a good idea to think of your brows—before you thin them, lighten them, or dye them—in relation to your dominant Station.

- If your First Station is dominant, emphasis should be upon the eyes, and the brows should not be too dark and heavy, or they will draw attention too much to the top of the face.

- If your Second Station is dominant, especially if you have a prominent nose, the brows should not be too light and thin, but should have good balance, and emphasis should be on both the eyes and the mouth to strengthen the weaker Stations.

- If your Third Section is dominant, strengthening the brows can draw attention away from a strong chin and bring your face into better balance.

When working with the brows, always keep in mind that they are your bridge between youth and maturity—your symbol of success as a person as well as your claim to fame. Don't neglect them—but don't let them dominate your face. Clear and well groomed, they show you care for yourself.

The Eyes—Intelligence

THE EYES ARE perhaps the most significant of the Five Major Features. They represent our inner energy—vitality, personality, and intelligence. The Position Points 35, 36, 37, 38, 39, and 40—the Yang and Yin Points—are in the eye itself. The ages covered by these points are often the most charismatic of a woman's life.

The eyes, luckily, are also the most adaptable feature when it comes to makeup; virtually any eye can be made to be beautiful with cosmetics. Further, beautiful eyes can be made to dominate the face, taking attention away from any other feature that is not so perfect. Beautiful eyes also diminish or take the attention away from minor or major signs of aging—so women in their late thirties do well to emphasize the eyes in their makeup and make the eyes the focus of the face.

In Chinese Face Reading, the left eye represents the sun (Yang, the male, or active characteristics) and the right eye the moon (Yin, the female, passive characteristics).

Some of the important characteristics of the eye cannot, of course, be modeled with makeup. The white of the eye should be white and clear. Occasional use of eyedrops can of course keep the white white if the eyes have been reddened from lack of sleep, too-bright light, and so on. However, the whiteness of the eye depends much on inner health; redness or yellowishness of the eyes is not considered fortunate or attractive. A tinge of blue on the white indicates a mystical nature.

The Chinese Face Readers also take into consideration the eyes' light. The ideal eye is brilliant, sparkles. The Chinese differentiate between this brilliance and the hectic too-bright glitter of eyes in one who is feverish or has taken certain drugs, such as barbiturates, which make the eyes unnaturally bright and wild. Another kind of unfavorable light is that noticed in the "roving" eye—of the sexually promiscuous person who always has an eye out for a new partner. Still another undesirable light is the wild or rolling eye of the person who is out of emotional control.

Desirable brilliance is that spark of intelligence, aliveness, and life force that catches another's eyes and truly attracts—the flash in the eyes of a Spanish dancer, the luminosity of those happily in love. Beautiful eye makeup brings out the sparkle in your eyes, as do good health and vitality. You can use a blue pencil to line the inner part of the lower lid (above the lashes) to make the eye seem brighter and the white of the eye whiter. Eyedrops also make the eyes seem brighter, but constant use should be avoided. Smiling inside and outside gives the eye sparkle; a controlled lust for life is also eye brightening. Dull eyes without sparkle denote poor health or a depressed, moody personality. The natural light of the eye can be used to command attention. Consider how you use your eyes. Keep them nicely open; move them when you talk but basically keep eye contact with the person with whom you are speaking. Draw attention with your eyes whenever and to whatever you choose. The use of the eyes is in itself an art.

THE IDEAL EYE

In Face Reading, the ideal eye is large, full and bright; the white is very white and clear. The person with such an eye is felt to be intelligent, courageous, artistic, sensitive, and capable of leadership.

When making up your eyes, you should try to get them to resemble this ideal eye—that is, to look as large, full, and open as possible; to be bright and sparkling and to reveal your animation and interest in life and people.

Because the basic eye makeup is so important and is much the same for any eye (for the various eye shapes, you make variations on this basic makeup) we give the basic makeup first and then go on to the characteristics of other eyes and how to make them appear large and luminous.

BASIC EYE MAKEUP

There are four basic eye-shadow areas:

1. The *underbrow highlight*. For the ideal eye, this is the lightest shade of the eye shadows. For evening it can be shimmering—ivory,

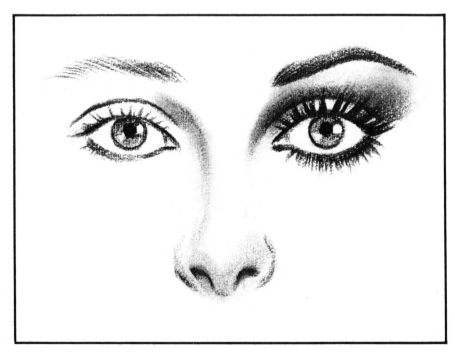

THE IDEAL EYE. When making up your eyes, try to get them to look large, full and open, bright, sparkling. This indicates intelligence, an interest in life.

gold and silver; for day, beige, light peach, light pink, or soft ivory. It is applied with a brush under the brow on the brow bone to reflect the light and make the space between the eye and the brow seem larger. Sometimes different shades of highlighter are placed on the inner eye bone, the middle and the outer for varying effect.

2. The *lid color* is the most interesting shadow. It is the "fashion" color and the brightest of the shadows. Its color should be coordinated with the color of the clothes you are wearing. The lid color is placed on the upper lid from the lashes to the crease in the upper lid. It may be a blend of three colors with the lightest in the inner third of the lid, the darkest at the outer third and the shiniest in the middle. For different eye effects, this can be varied.

3. The *contour* is the darkest of the shadows and is used to enhance the eye's three-dimensional appearance. Apply it with a small-tip brush or crayon. Start the contour above the crease in the upper lid and bring it slightly up so that it is visible when the eye is open and looking straight ahead. It can be fanned out slightly toward the outer tip of the eye. The contour color should be cocoa, gray, ginger, smoky blue or green, or any brown tone.

4. Shadow is used below the eye toward the *outer tip* to round the shape of the eye. It can be in the lid color or in the contour color. Apply lightly, blend to be as smooth as possible.

Eye Liner

Liner defines the shape of the eye if used softly, but will close the eye in and make it look smaller if it is too dark or too heavy. Don't try to change the shape of the eye. Just follow the contour of the upper lid as close to the lashes as possible. Use a soft taupe or brown liner, if any, in daytime so it doesn't dominate the eye. For evening, colored liner is best—blue, green, navy, or charcoal. Liner can also be used on the lower lid, right in the lower lashes, very fine, but do not go all the way to the inner corner of the eye. Instead, start about a third of the way across and draw the line lightly right in the lashes following the shape of the eye to the outer tip.

If you want to put a blue liner on the lower lid above the lashes for evening, hold the lower lid down and, with a blue pencil, draw the line along the top of the lower lid just above the lashes. (Do not get the pencil on the inside of the eye or it will be irritating.) This will make the white of the eye seem brighter and the eyes more luminous.

Mascara

Mascara is the finishing touch that makes your eyes totally lovely. To apply effectively, coat both the bottom and top lashes, rolling the applicator as you apply. The applicator both feeds mascara onto the lashes and brushes them so that they are separated as you roll the applicator over them. Do the upper side of the upper lashes first. When they are dry do the undersides. Next, do the undersides of the lower lashes, picking up the lashes individually with the applicator wand. When the lashes are dry, do the upper sides of the lower lashes. Use your finger underneath the lashes as you apply mascara to keep the mascara off the skin. When all lashes are dry, brush for further separation.

Soft black or brown mascara can be used in daytime; black, blue, navy, emerald, purple for evening.

Application

When applying eye makeup, keep both eyes equally open at all times. Tilt the head back and look in the mirror or use a mirror flat on the dressing table and look down into it. The lids should be relaxed. To apply liner, rest the heel of the hand high against the cheek and use the little finger as a pivot; apply liner with little light strokes, working from the inner tip of the lid outward. If you tend to make a heavier line when you start, work from the middle of the eye inward and then outward to the outer tip of the eye.

EYE MAKEUP STEP-BY-STEP

Here is the order of doing your eye makeup no matter what your eye shape or size:

1. Start with a crease-resistant base or a coating of translucent powder all over the eye area to prevent streaking. Apply with a brush from the upper lashes to the brows and around the entire eye.

2. Do the highlighter next—the lighest shadow shade—above the crease to the brows over the brow bone.

3. Then do lid colors. Apply the basic color all over the bottom half of the upper lid to the crease, and then a lighter color at the inner corner and a highlighter in the middle. NOTE: This sequence is for the ideal eye. See below how to vary the applications of lid colors for your particular eye shape.

4. Now the contour—the deepest shadow shade. This goes above the crease in the upper lid, brushed upward toward the brow bone and slightly outward toward the temple at the outer tip of the lid.

5. Blend the edges of the three shadows together so that they merge into each other, but do not blur the colors.

6. Apply shadow if needed below the eye at the outer edge of the lower lid and extend upward to fan into the contour shadow at the outer tip. Blend into the contour line.

7. Line upper lid lash line and outer half of the lower lid.

8. Mascara tops and bottoms of both upper and lower lashes.

VARIATIONS ON EYES

The eyes should be the focus point of the face. The ideal eyes are wide and large and open, well placed on the face in relation to other features, and with lots of the upper lid showing (this is a protection for the eyes). The white should be white, the irises (colored part of the eyes) bright, and the eyes should reflect a controlled light. If you have this kind of eye, you impress others with your intelligence, capacity for leadership, harmonious personality, and your feminine power. The makeup given above is designed for the ideal eye, but you may need to modify it only slightly to bring out the most beautiful qualities of other eyes.

1. Large Full Eyes

This is close to the ideal eye—and it says you are intelligent, sensitive, artistic. Others feel that you are open and frank. You can succeed in positions of leadership, in the theater, and the other arts, for you are an excellent observer and naturally outgoing. You may not, however, be happy as a homemaker because you want to be out seeing things and sharing experiences. These eyes attract sexual partners easily— for eyes are an erotic feature and one of the first things that you notice about others—but you may suffer disappointments in love, partly because you attract men too easily as your eyes are always attention getters.

You can follow the makeup steps for the ideal eye, because your eyes are not really a problem. However, be sure to keep the space between your eyes and brow as wide as possible and carefully define the brow arch to frame your eyes, keeping the brows fairly thick. Emphasize the lids with three shades of translucent shadows on the lid—deeper on the outer half of the upper lid, lighter on the inner part of the lid, with a highlight in the middle. Extend shadow at the outer tip of the lid to make the eye more luminous. Use a deep color in the contour area (above the crease) to emphasize your eyes' fullness and size.

As you will be using your eyes to extend the range of your experience, do not be shy about makeup but be skillful and neat about how you apply it. Your artistic qualities help you become an expert

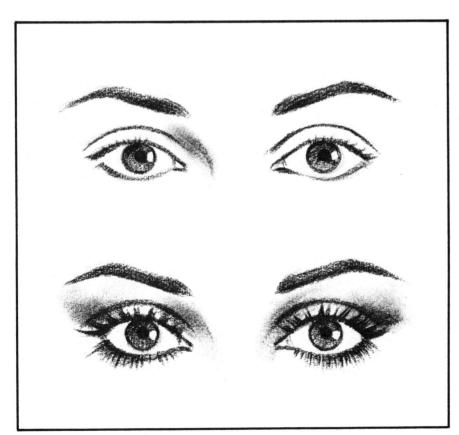

LARGE FULL EYES. Too much heavy makeup on these eyes can diminish their shape rather than open them up. Use a deep color in the contour area to emphasize fullness. The owner of these eyes is naturally outgoing.

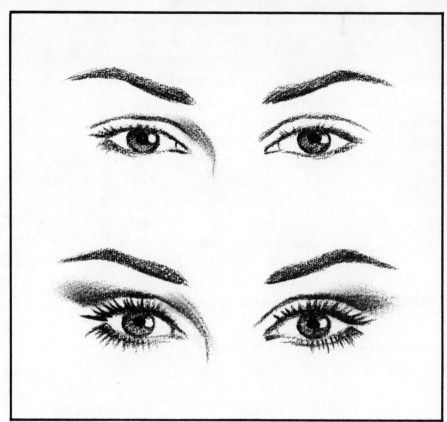

SMALL EYES.
Dark liner will only
shut these eyes in.
Use a light liner
and extend it slightly
at the tail of the eyes.
These eyes indicate
self-satisfaction,
introspection.

makeup artist—at least on yourself. Your eyes may be your most attractive feature, so make the most of them. Too much heavy makeup on a full eye can diminish its shape rather than open it up.

2. *Small Eyes*

Small eyes indicate someone who is loyal in relationships, methodical but perhaps complacent about her skills and abilities. To be considered small your eyes should be small in comparison to the rest of the features on your face, so consider carefully whether they really are small or merely deep-set. It is possible, because you tend not to be pushy—in fact, you may be very self-satisfied and introspective and not inclined to make the most of your face—that you may not do everything you can to make your eyes attractive. Others then tend to consider you hard to get to know—even unapproachable—and won't make the effort. In the long run, this may mean you won't develop your talents,

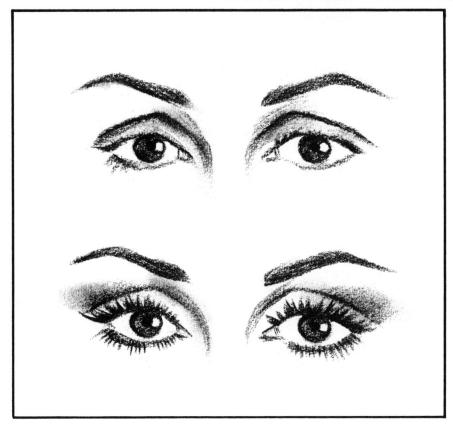

DEEP-SET EYES. Keep the brow very high and arched to give more open space to the eyes. With these eyes, one is likely to be a dreamer, intelligent but conservative.

and you do have them. Many painters and those with talents in other artistic fields have small eyes; so do students and experts in many areas. You also tend to have strong moral standards, and are not easily won over into a relationship. Once someone has your heart, he can expect you to be devoted and steadfast and to be very supportive. Alas, you tend to be jealous—perhaps because you feel you don't have the assets other women have. Start by making more of your eyes, for this can be the start of self-confidence. It will also incline those who can use your talents to be more aware and receptive to your abilities so that the door of opportunity will be opened wider. So don't sit there squinting. These simple makeup tricks will give you a bright-eyed look and you'll feel more congenial to everybody.

· First, raise your eyebrows; keep your brow thin, high and pale in color so that there is more space around the eye for you to work with.

- The highlight under the brow should be very light and reflect a soft pale glow.

- On your lids, use the palest of bright colors—light green, blue, or light gray-blue—to put the emphasis on and enlarge the lid area. Bring the color all the way to the crease. This will make the upper lid more prominent by reflecting light. A highlight on the middle of the upper lid will also be light-catching.

- Use a medium-shade contour color and, starting above the crease, bring it as high as you can above the lid to lift the whole eye area— even as high as the socket bone above the eye.

- Liner should expand the eye—the softer and brighter the color, the better. Colors are better than neutrals for this eye. All shadows should be coordinated in the same color scheme, so the eyes become more evident and exciting.

- Use shadow under the eye for a slightly smudged look, or use a soft undereye liner for a rounding effect.

- Don't try to enlarge the eye with dark liner, because you will only close the eye in. You can use light liner and extend the liner slightly at the tail of the eye—but don't make it too emphatic.

Because you tend to encapsulate life, view it, so to speak, on a small screen, you find it easy to do everything beautifully—as some of those who work on a larger canvas do not. You can become very clever with your eye makeup and do something to particularly enhance your eyes. The period when you are in the late thirties, emphasizing the qualities denoted by the eyes, may not be an expansive time for you, but it is likely to be an age when you get everything exactly the way you want it and will have the right to feel very smug about your achievement.

3. Deep-Set Eyes

With these eyes you are likely to be a dreamer, more romantic than passionate, more intellectual than physical, but remarkably good in money matters. As you tend to be a thinker, you are rarely impulsive and always somewhat conservative in your approach. You do not often take chances. But because you dream and have romantic fantasies, you may be an easier prey than you'd like to the male charmer who recognizes your sensitive qualities and wants to make you his captive—temporarily. With your deep-set eyes you are both trustful and can be trusted, and so are easily hurt. Look carefully for the stable qualities in those to whom you confide yourself so that you will not be misled. In your late thirties, you may be inclined to be too introspective—just at a period when you should be making your impact on the world. But if you have turned your fantasies into actualities, your dreams into realities, you will be sought after for your inner wisdom.

· In makeup your deep-set eyes need to be brought out to reveal their sparkle and color and intelligent charm. Usually, with deep-set eyes, the brow bone is very prominent. Keep the brow very high and arched to give more open space to the eyes.

· As the bone area is high, do not follow the usual pattern of putting a highlight on this area. Instead use a *warm* color on the bone beneath the brow—peach, warm rich beige, a light ginger—all over the brow-bone area so it will not stand out too much.

· The lid color should be light—the lightest of blue, green, gray, or ivory, and you should stick to the cool colors, avoiding the warm earth tones here.

· The contour color should be *bright* because this crease in the lid is often naturally deep. Fan it out in a triangular shape at the outer edge of the eye, to lift the corner of the eye up and to overcome any droop in this area.

· Use a medium color under the eye—never very dark. A bright liner, starting under the iris and going toward the outer part of the eye, also opens the eye. Leave the inner corner open and unlined.

Because your deep-set eyes give you financial skills, you are likely to be an asset to anyone with whom you enter into a partnership, and also to provide intelligent care for yourself. Avoid a tendency to narrow your eyes too much when thinking or to let them half close when you feel introspective; increase your options by holding eye contact with those with whom you speak.

4. Protruding Eyes

You are a gambler by nature and always have an eye out for a deal—and tend also to gamble with people and be indulgent sexually. But you are also ambitious and strong minded and not at all the wastrel that others might suppose. With this eye, you tend to be extroverted—to live in the outer world much more than in the inner world—and this may make you at times rash and impulsive. You tend to make easy changes in your life—because you are so willing to take chances—and in the years between thirty-five and forty, when the matters pertaining to the eye are emphasized, you will find out how well this gambling has paid off. As you have a powerful will of your own and know what you want, you most likely will have made considerable waves and reached a dominant position at this middle period. Don't be surprised, however, if you suddenly risk everything once again. You will be confident in your own strength, but others may be uneasy if their welfare is closely tied to yours. Protruding eyes command attention and you are likely to look people in the eye and get control over them with your glance. It's very important esthetically that these eyes be balanced with other features of the face.

- Avoid rounded eyebrows. You need a more standard arched brow that cuts down at an angle to modify the roundness of the eye.

- Keep the highlighter in a medium color, warm but not too light.

- The lid color should be smoky—earth-oriented—to reduce the appearance of the large lid and avoid a bulging look. Cocoa, gray, ginger, and claret are very good.

- You need a definite contour in basic dark tones—deep cocoa, deep navy, deep brown.

- Liner should be slightly deeper brown or soft black. Line above and below to frame the whole eye and so reduce its size. Use an underliner in a smoky color, avoiding all lights around the eye.

- Lining the whole eye helps it seem less protruding; emphasize the middle eye with extra mascara on the middle lashes of the upper and lower lid.

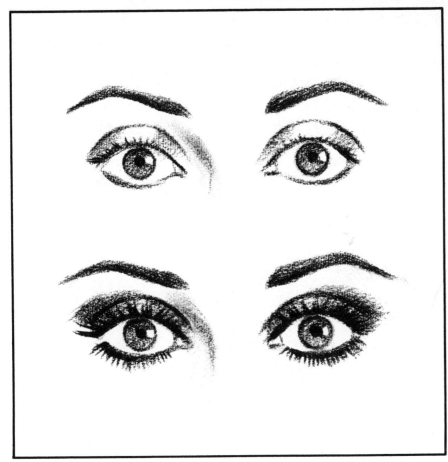

PROTRUDING EYES. Lining the whole eye makes it seem less bulging. Use extra mascara on the middle lashes of both lids. These are the eyes of a gambler —but one who is strong-minded and ambitious.

Because your eyes are noticeable and usually bright because they catch the light, try to avoid negative habits, such as rolling the eyes and focusing anywhere other than on the eyes of the person with whom you are speaking. You can comfortably let your lids drop a little instead of striving for a wide-eyed look. As your eyes tend to speak of your own earthy feelings, you'll understand why men so often follow you and so many try to pick you up and generally consider you inviting. Your problem is that others may think you're superficial —when you actually have a firm idea of what you want from life for yourself, and will take all sorts of chances to get it. If other features back your eyes up, you succeed in enterprises where some risk taking is a part of the game. You don't need to play it safe in relationships or in a career. And in a tight corner, you can always spot a way out.

5. *Upturned Eyes*

This is a cheerful eye. Those looking at you expect you to be fun—optimistic, brave, and a bit of an adventurer. And you are. You also are likely to be opportunistic, decisive and self-confident, but often very short-tempered and likely not to hold back. You are quick witted—a trait that is very useful in a variety of enterprises. You catch on to what is needed at any moment and have ideas and carry them out handily. Especially, you are someone great to be around because your enthusiasm is catching and you're into exciting things and take chances with a true adventurous spirit. You do, though, tend to have short-term goals and like things to happen fast and enjoy changes. To use your quick intelligence, perky personality, and superconfidence best, get into a job where you have to make quick decisions, where there is plenty of action and others as well as you are on the move. As an emotional partner you are likely to be unreasonable, impatient and jealous, and your violent temper will be disruptive—even if your tantrums quickly pass. You probably won't rock the boat in an emergency—you're too quick-thinking for that. But you might rock it in calm waters—just to see some action—and this can be equally hazardous. Because you take advantage of every situation to help yourself first and because you are not afraid to venture into shaky situations, you probably will come into your late thirties with a lot of self-confidence and with your career pretty well made. You aren't afraid of changes, so this may be a period when you will change again—forever light-hearted and confident that you'll get what you want. And you will.

Because the uptilted eye is an attractive, young-looking eye, there is no reason to do much to change it—especially if you are using its characteristics in a positive fashion. If you do change it, do so only slightly.

- If you want your eyes to look rounder and larger and less uptilted, follow the basic makeup. But on the lid, use more opaque color in the inner corner, and sheerer color at the outer corner.

- Use more liner at the inner corner and taper the line to nothing at the outer corner.

- Use a softer under line, starting at the middle of the eye and going

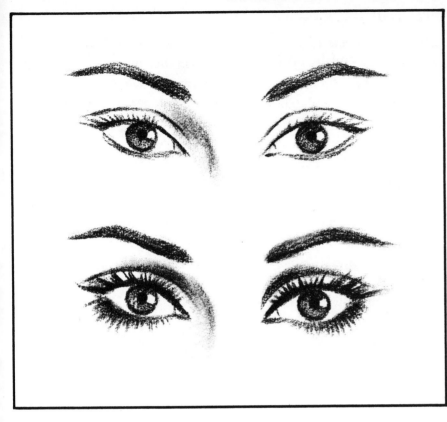

UPTURNED EYES. Line the inner corner and taper the line to nothing at the outer tip, with just a smudge of shadow under the outer tip. These eyes indicate you are quick-witted —and short-tempered.

to the outer end, and leave the inner corner open. Make just a slight smudge of shadow under the eye at the *outer* tip. This makes the eye larger, rounder, less upswept.

With these cheerful, self-confident eyes, you don't need heavy makeup or dark colors. Keep your makeup simple and clean, especially for day and for your encounters in the business world. You are someone people like to pal with, run with, have fun with, for they seem to pick up your natural vitality. You can use more eye makeup at night, when you are likely to feel more teasing, emotional and exotic—and then this adventurer's eyes can be haunting and mysterious. Your chief problem is that the eyes reflect intelligence—and you are at times totally unreasonable. You have to rely on your quick-wittedness to overcome a tendency not to be reasonable at all when your will is thwarted. If you use your qualities in a positive fashion, you can grasp all the great opportunities that will be offered you.

6. Down-Turned Eyes

If the outer corners of your eyes are at a lower level than the inner corners, so the eye droops at the end, your eyes may seem sad. You are likely to be self-effacing and considerate of others. But being so pleasant, you are likely to be submissive to the opposite sex and easily victimized. Your intelligence is of the humanitarian sort—you understand others' dilemmas but may not be able to deal easily with your own, because the sad look of your eyes makes you feel dependent, undermining your self-confidence and occupying your mind with the superficial and immediate problems of life. This could result in a kind of soap-opera existence, in which you reel from problems of your own to those of others (so quick are you to lend a helping hand, even if it pulls you down into the morass in the process) and back to your own misadventures, so that you never really set up a direction and goal that could be your salvation. This is particularly true if you also have droopy brows—but the two do not always go together. One way to offset this victim psychology is to modify your eyes with makeup so they look less sad, and put you into a better mood. As you gain confidence, others have more respect for you, and you are helped to achievement.

- Contour but little on the inner corner of the eye and use a heavier contour at the outer corner, almost as for deep-set eyes (above).

- When using eye liner, leave the inner corner open and start the line under the inner side of the iris (as you look straight ahead), and extend the eye line at the outer corner slightly, bringing it out and straight up.

- Do the undereye liner close to the inner corner and taper it toward the outer corner.

- Apply the lid shadow in the same way, with little in the inner corner and a translucent shadow on the outer half of the lid, extending it slightly up.

- With a droopy eye, avoid a flared or uptilted brow. The ideal regular arch is better, but neither lift the arch too much nor let the outer tip come down too far.

If you have a down-slanted eye, you may cry easily and this could be a handicap in coping with problems—or an asset. Some men melt when a woman cries. You do better, however, if you stiffen your confidence and rely on the pleasant aspects of your nature to win your points. Many fields are open to those who are pleasant and ingratiating, as you are, and understand others' problems. You may not want too much responsibility (unless other features on your face create strength), but all the fields requiring patience and sympathy—nursing, social work, settling complaints, working with the handicapped —require emotional intelligence. And realize, too, you need not always be a victim; sad eyes evoke pity, and people want to help you. If nature gave you a voice and a sense of show business, sad eyes are an asset to a blues singer. If you are skillful with your hands, your compassion is welcome in arts and crafts where love is transferred to objects. In your personal relationships, your natural dependence may be an asset, for a man will want to take care of you if you find the right one. If you've had several faulty relationships by the time you're

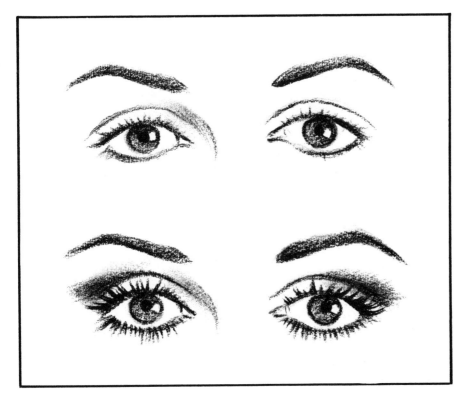

DOWN-TURNED EYES. Leave the inner corner of the eye open and emphasize the outer corner with a heavier contour liner. Avoid a flared or uptilted browline. With these eyes, you are likely to be self-effacing, considerate of others.

thirty-five, this may be the time (emphasized by the eyes) when you are at last able to find someone as kind and thoughtful and in need of loving as you are.

7. *Large Eye with Small Iris*

In Face Reading this is called the "three-white-sided eye," because the white of the eye is visible under the iris (the colored part of the eye) as well as at the sides. Such an eye makes its owner look in danger all the time, and indicates someone who is temperamental and as a result often appears menacing. In fact, if you have such an eye you must guard against being unscrupulous, even cruel in a crunch, because you can alienate others. It's possible you will be discontented with many of the circumstances in your life and rebel against restrictions, because you tend to take a rather narrow view of things and are basically restless. Others may feel you are unreliable and it may be difficult for you to establish yourself for both these reasons—your own tendency not to get along with the team and the fears of your colleagues that you will prove unreliable. It may be a good idea for you to accept only short-term commitments, so you won't have time to get bored and restless—and so that you will forever get what you need in life: a fresh start. Study the better features of your face, and work with those to overcome any deficiency in your inner energy, which is clearly erratic. In personal relationships you need lots of chances to "vacation" from your mate to restore this inner energy through entertainment breakaways. Avoid people who try to pin you down, and seek out those who are oriented to diversions. On the positive side you are likely to be generous. But you have a tendency to lose things and are careless with money. Many different people will seek you out, because a lot of white showing in the eyes is considered a kind of come-on. These people may not always be wholesome sorts. As the small iris makes you somewhat shrewd, you can evaluate them fairly well. Your own restlessness, though, tempts you into casual, often careless, relationships.

You can protect yourself by modifying your eyes somewhat to make a better impression and to give you protection from those who too often will prey upon your weaknesses.

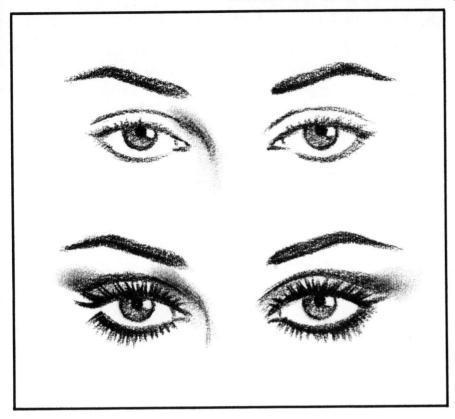

LARGE EYE WITH SMALL IRIS. Shadow and contouring should be in shades of one color—in different degrees of intensity. Use lots of liner, thicker in the middle, to modify upper lid; a strong underliner. These eyes show restlessness.

- As the upper lid is often straight and the lower lid rounded, the shadow and contouring on the eye should be all in one color—in monochromatic colors but in different degrees of intensity. Use lots of liner, thicker in the middle to create roundness in the upper lid, and a strong underliner to detract from the white.

- A blue or gray line on the lower lid above the lashes closes in the lower lid—so there will seem less white of the eye in focus. Other than that, you can follow the makeup for the ideal eye, with the modifications for the large eye.

As the age span of the late thirties focuses on the eyes, a crisis of temperament due to erratic inner energy may develop about them. Try to develop the stronger parts of your nature to overcome the restlessness that will perhaps beset you.

HOW YOUR EYES ARE SET

The eyes' position on the face and their size both play an important part in the balance of the face. If eyes are set too close together it indicates too much dependence on parents and a consequently narrow point of view in self-development. If eyes are disproportionately wide apart, it can show some separation between the parents or parental influence. The first is a sign of a person who tends to weakness; the second of one who may become too strong. If eyes are properly balanced, it shows one who is adjusted to society and in harmony with the world.

Close-set Eyes

• If eyes are close-set, extend shadow out at the outer corner. Use a light color on the inner half of the lid and a brighter color on the outer half, extending the color slightly beyond the length of the lid, and blend where the colors meet.

• Start the liner two thirds of the way in on the upper lid and again extend slightly at the outer corner.

• Use two applications of highlighter—the inner half very light and the outer medium.

• If you wear glasses, keep the frame color light at the bridge and at the inner sides of the frame, and avoid a heavy or intricate bridge.

Widely-spaced Eyes

For these eyes, the emphasis is just the opposite. Widely-spaced eyes give an impression of strength and youth and innocence and there is usually no particular reason to make them any different.

• However, if you desire better balance, put more color on the inner part of the eye and a softer color on the outer part. Don't extend the shadow at the end of the eye or bring it close to the inner corner of the upper lid.

• On the lower lid, line very close to the inner corner. Come all the way in, following the full length of the eye.

· Eyeglasses with a strong bridge and dark color in the middle part of the frame make eyes seem closer together.

OTHER EYE FACTORS

A Lot of White Showing

This indicates one who is accident prone. With white showing above and below the pupil, it indicates one who has a wild temper and may actually become violent when angry. (Someone to avoid in a singles' bar.)

The Color of the Irises

If the iris is dark brown, it indicates vitality; blue eyes are bright and happy natured; green eyes are more mysterious and intellectual; violet eyes are exceptionally charismatic. Yellow pupils show one is temperamental.

Lashes

If lashes are long, it shows one who is soft-hearted, sensitive, spiritual, and not at all mean and aggressive. Short thick lashes show a doer, someone who *is* strong and aggressive, If lashes are thin and loose, it denotes inactivity, perhaps poor circulation.

Laugh Lines

Many laugh lines (crow's feet) at the corner of the eye show sexual indulgence (especially in a man). If the crow's feet point upward, one is a self-achiever. If the crow's feet go down, it indicates divorce.

Thick Lids

These indicate a sensuous nature, strongmindedness.

SPECIAL EYES

· If you wear contact lenses, use no powder shadow, no lash-lengthening mascara; instead choose a cream shadow; waterproof mascara. This saves you from specks of cosmetics behind your lenses.

- If you wear eyeglasses, emphasize eye makeup. Use *more* makeup and in brighter or deeper colors, and even stronger eyeliner to define the eyes. If lashes beat against your eyeglasses lenses, curl the lashes with a lash curler as high as possible before putting on mascara.

- If you are a mature woman and your eyelid skin tends to be crinkly, avoid powder eye makeup and frosted shadows because these emphasize the texture of the eye skin. Matte cream shadows are a better choice.

- Black women should avoid matte-finish makeup on the eyes as it tends to make the skin look ashen. As your skin tone is rich and your features often tend to be dramatic, you can use dramatic colors and glistening shadows. Frosted shadows are wonderful for you because they tend to be lighter and let the skin color show through. Matte shadows give too much coverage and look too heavy.

- If you are a very young teenager, avoid heavy dramatic eye colors. Choose skin-related colors in a transparent form.

EYE POSITION POINTS

These are very interesting. Points 33 and 34—the areas beneath the brows where we usually apply our highlighter—represent "rainbows." Point 33 on the right eye represents a colorful rainbow—light refracted into its natural array of colors from deep violet to infrared as it is in a rainbow in the sky. Point 34 on the left lid represents a kaleidoscope of color—color broken into random parts as it might be in disco lighting or by prisms. Obviously, if these are your present Position Points (ages 32–33), they represent a colorful period in your life. For those who work with color—artists, decorators, painters, photographers, dressmakers, cosmetic people—these are significant points to observe for their quality and indications of how you fare at present in the natural color scheme. Points 37 and 38—the pupils of the eye—represent, respectively, middle Yin and middle Yang. Yin (feminine, passive) and Yang (masculine, active) are the negative and positive forces of the universe. Your inner energy is expressed through these points. As these points are in the pupils—where reflected light creates the sparkle—they are significant of vitality.

The eyes are Star Points. The years of life represented by the Position Points of the eyes are times when you star.

Because of this significance of the eye, you can hardly ever go wrong if you make the eyes the focus of the face.

The Nose—Wealth

THE NOSE represents money—your ability to seek out opportunity, to accumulate wealth (or to waste it). Its Position Points (41 to 50) represent the decade of the forties—the prime of life where you establish yourself in career, profession, or business. The nose is a "mountain"—a high point of the face—and a large and impressive nose is in actuality a key to success and wealth. Before you decide you "hate your nose," consider what it can mean to your life pattern.

The area between the eyes is called Moon Dust. It is a Star Point and the Palace of Health. Position Point 41, the Root of the Mountain, is a health point. But this area is also the seat or start of your climb in the world of business. If it is clear and smooth and of good color, you will have clear sailing. If it is rough or lumpy, or if it has a horizontal line across it, you may have a rough start in the business world—and also domestic difficulties, for this point also affects your destiny with your marriage partner and family. One crosswise line here indicates you'll leave home early. Two lines here on a man's nose is a warning that he will be hard on his wife and family—perhaps by being too critical, too demanding, too self-centered, a drifter. In a woman's face, this horizontal line is an indicator of the same tendencies, but it is somewhat less potentially dangerous to the husband, because he so often holds the reins of power in the household and business. Three transverse lines mean you'll accomplish much by your own efforts. If you have a vertical line down the nose, it indicates you'll adopt children.

If the Root of the Mountain is hollow, it can adversely affect your health and longevity as well as your success in business and marriage.

If it is flat and broad, it indicates an ability to create a warm, happy family life; if high, it gives promise of strength in work and family and a long, rich life as well.

To each side of the nose at the inner corners of the eye lie Position Points 42 and 43—which indicate the kind of home you will have—and this age (41, 42) is a time in life when many people do buy a house or change residences. Point 42 on the left side of the nose indicates a Delicate Cottage or hideaway, so it may also indicate a time when you want to escape and restore your inner strength. Point 43 is a Bright Parlor—a kind of entertainment center or "court," indicating a great many guests and an outgoing kind of social life for this period.

Points 44 and 45 on the bridge of the nose have much to do with your health as well as your success. As physical and emotional and mental vitality are a great factor in success in business, you can see how these points are influential.

Point 44 is literally translated as Sitting on Top of One's Age. As in Western terms age forty-three is related to the start of the midlife crisis, when you come to terms with the fact that you aren't a young chick any more and assume the vitalities and gifts of the prime of life, it is a point at which you move ahead or drop back. Point 45, related to your health, is Sitting on Top of One's Longevity. This is an "age point'" (44 years) when many people give up their destructive habits, and marshal the resources of healthful living for a rich full life ahead.

Points 46 and 47 are on the cheekbones and relate to your power, which also affects your moneymaking ability and the chance to realize career ambitions at this time of life. But 48 at the tip of the nose is the most significant point. It represents the "peak of perfection"—the acme of your success. It reflects the culmination of your middle years. The area of the tip of the nose is the Palace of Wealth. And a strong well-rounded tip can assure you of success. Positions 49 and 50 on the nostrils represent the manner in which your personality affects your success. If the nostrils are full and flared you are likely to be outgoing; if thin and pinched, you may be miserly and moneygrubbing. They also show how you deal with the success you have achieved at the peak of perfection—whether you hang onto it or dissipate it.

Of course you have your nose all your life—and have to live with it in your teens, twenties and thirties, no matter what it promises you for later on. The ideal nose is smooth and well formed at the root (for a good start in career by a stable family life); it has a smooth full area at Points 42 and 43 for comfortable living conditions; the bridge should be straight (Points 44, 45) for good health and vitality and a chance to live long to develop one's capacity. If the nose is flat in this area, you have to work hard all your life to make a living. The tip (Point 48) should be well rounded and the whole line of the nose should be well formed from base to tip, with nostril wings rounded and slightly flared. With this ideal nose, a person can expect achievement in life and to enjoy honors, wealth, and good family and friends.

As we've seen, the nose by its nature should be prominent—it should stand out from the face. Unfortunately, more women are dissatisfied with their noses than with any other features—because, of course, it *does* stand out. It is difficult to change the prominent nose with makeup—although some subtle things can be done. You can also balance a prominent nose with your hairdo and the makeup of eyes and mouth, your earrings, neckline and other accessories so that it blends into the face with greater harmony.

The nose is, nevertheless, the feature most often being changed by cosmetic surgery—and particularly among teenage girls, who are especially anxious at that age about their looks. Here, a word of warning. Till puberty (early teens) the individual has a child's nose—its mature shape does not begin to develop until the sexual organs develop. The nose, itself, is considered a sexual organ because of the powerful impact our sense of smell has upon our emotions. But the nose doesn't reach its full maturity till age twenty or twenty-one. As the development of the nose is clearly related to the maturing and development of the brain, it is very unwise to submit it to surgery until it is well developed and completely mature. The rest of the face is still developing, too. The chin does not really mature in a woman until the late twenties. You may, in fact, be less than satisfied with your nose job if it is done too early. A nose job often involves an adjustment in the chin or lower jaw to balance the new feature. If you feel you must make a surgical change in any feature, wait till your face is completely mature.

Some of the least liked characteristics for beauty in the nose are the most desirable for success in career and family life. In fact, the thin bony nose that is considered the ideal for beauty is *not* the ideal for happiness and success. If too thin through the bridge, it is known as the "widow's nose"—the mark of someone who is hard on her husband(s) and may end up lonely and dissatisfied.

Although the nose does more than any other major feature to give "character" to the face (as the eyes and brows give charisma), and is the most elevated feature, it still is not much noticed by others. Listen to descriptions of missing persons or wrongdoers—you hear about the color of the hair and eyes, what the person was wearing, how tall or short, how thick or thin, but no one ever tells you anything about the person's nose. Try to call up the shape of the nose of people you know or see on television—except for those who've made a big thing of their nose (Streisand, Bob Hope)—it's just not something you remember. The nose you hate may be less noticeable than you think. On the other hand, cartoonists who want to exaggerate the character of a face will nearly always exaggerate the shape and size of the nose to give an instant caricature.

NOSE SHAPES AND HOW TO CORRECT THEM

1. Straight Nose

This nose promises you financial success. You are honest, even-tempered, enterprising, and can reach a high position in life. This will partly be due to good health and vitality, a stable family life, and a long life in which to achieve your goals. If you have this kind of nose, it is wise to call attention to it—by giving a prospective employer or business partner or personal companion a chance to view it in profile and by keeping it well lifted and, so to speak, on display. If you have such a nose, people are going to admire you and trust you, because they believe you are in your nature straight and honest and will never play dirty tricks.

Cosmetically, there is little you have to do with this nose, except to observe its color. The nose should have a peachy glow. If your nose doesn't have this color, is too pale or too pink, it will benefit from a little color on the tip. Use a faint brush of peach-glow blusher.

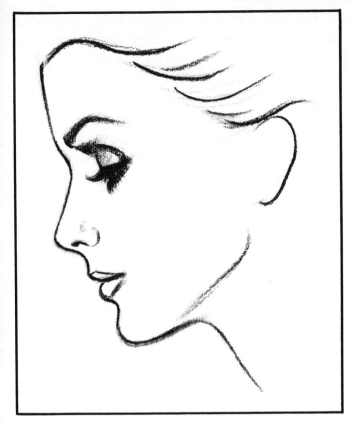

STRAIGHT NOSE.
This nose promises financial success—
an honest nature. It needs no correction
—except possibly for color: a faint
peach blush if it is pale or too pink.

One thing you have to consider: Though this is a successful nose, and a financially good nose, it is an "ethical" nose. You aren't cut out for businesses and professions where values are compromised and deals are made behind closed doors and under the table. Get into work or a profession where "values" are respected.

2. Bony Nose

A thin bony nose, often with a sharp tip, although regarded as aristocratic and the nose of beauty, indicates arrogance and excess pride. It's owner is likely to be excessively self-centered, and very often alone because she is naturally hypercritical and a perfectionist. If you have this kind of nose, you probably like to live alone—no one else messing up your life—and especially to work alone, because no one else does things as well as you do. In fact, if you insist on being arrogant, you will probably find it hard to discover anyone who will work for you very long or who will live with you very long. If you have enough money to live on—and you often do because you've inherited it or have had a lucrative marriage settlement or have just saved it up—you do best to gratify your solitary self-centered needs. Of course, other features on your face may indicate quite different traits, and grant you favors and successes in other ways; your brows may bring you fame, your cheekbones give you power, your sensual mouth may attract lovers.

You can also modify your nose with makeup so that it will impress others as being more warm and friendly. This is, however, a highly technical kind of makeup and takes a lot of practice and skill. You probably shouldn't attempt it except for evening and then only for special public appearances. But as you are likely to be careful with details, you may manage it very well.

With a slightly lighter foundation—and this is only one or two shades of color-change different from your regular foundation—make a somewhat wide line from the top of the nose all the way to the tip. Use your regular darker foundation on the sides of the nose and a slightly lighter shade in the indentations of the nostril flares at the sides of the nose. If the tip of the nose is sharp, use a little peachy blusher on the tip to make it appear more rounded.

As the characteristics of this nose become more pronounced in the forties, you should prepare yourself in your earlier years to make adjustments to loneliness and possibly discontent that may confront you then. You are demanding, want to rule and like to be waited upon, so get into a field where you can be in control.

3. Aquiline Nose

This is Cleopatra's nose. Blaise Pascal said that if it had been one inch shorter, the face of the world would have been changed—perhaps meaning that the famous queen of Egypt would not have been so quick to enter into sexual relations with her conquerors, that she would have had less sagacity and power in dealing with the Romans. Anyone with this nose tends to be sexy—even oversexed—and also to have a good business sense, to be shrewd, even crafty, streetwise, and selfish. These are all useful characteristics for today's businesswoman. For many successful women in industry and business, it has been a nose for money, a nose for power and a nose for fascinating rich hus-

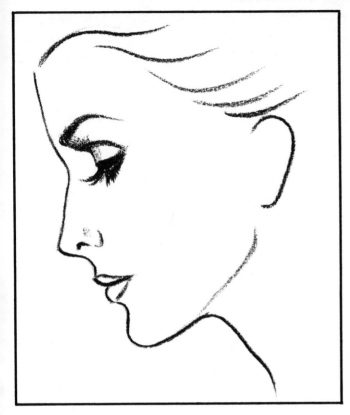

BONY NOSE.
If the tip of the nose is sharp, use a little
peach blusher on the tip to round it
out. This is the nose of beauty but it
may also indicate arrogance and
pride—a perfectionist.

bands. You also probably have an exceedingly good sense of smell. A famous "nose" of the perfume business, Prince Matchabelli, the creator of expensive glamorous perfumes, also had this nose. If it is yours, you will probably be able to choose the scent that does most to surround you with an aura of sensuality and success. In fact, so many attributes of achievement and wealth go with this nose that many successful women wear it proudly and would not think of changing its shape. Others find it too masculine and prominent and it is frequently bobbed.

If you want to keep your nose but deemphasize its shrewdness, a little dark foundation under the tip can make it appear shorter.

As this is a businesswoman's nose, it shouldn't interfere with your success in life—except that those planning to go into business with you may fear your competition or think you are smarter than they. Emphasize your eyes, surround yourself with your sexy scent, and they will fail to notice how acquisitive your nose is.

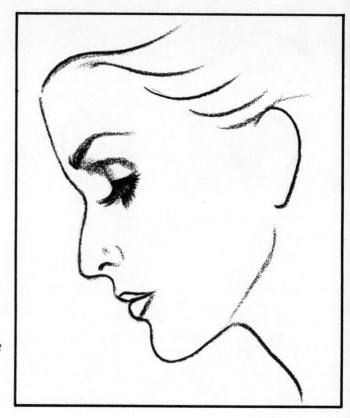

AQUILINE NOSE.
A little dark foundation under the tip
can make this nose appear shorter. It is
a nose for money, for power and for
fascinating rich husbands. Achievement
and wealth go with this nose.

4. Short Nose

The short nose is often cute, youthful, fun. It shows that you are open minded, optimistic, and outgoing—and have a strong impulse to share your enthusiasms with others. In fact, with this nose you have to guard against being sexually promiscuous, overemotional, too impulsive. This nose is not going to give you a powerful career, and it is not going to help you accumulate a lot of money. But it does give you a cheerful outlook and you have no trouble finding helpers, because you're energetic and fun to be around. You are probably not going to be too ambitious and will happily work for short-term goals, feeling tomorrow will take care of itself—and you can always find some way to get along. Employers like to take you on because you are cheerful and look honest and good hearted and feel you will work well with other people—which you do. You can also adjust easily to changes and are not at all judgmental—taking people as they are and making the best of situations that arise. You also have a short interest span—

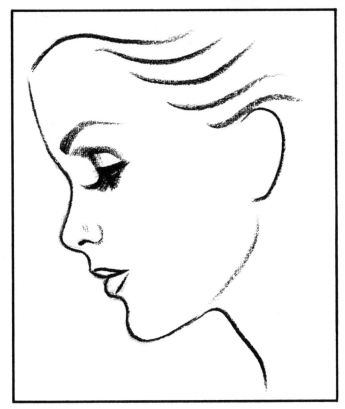

SHORT NOSE.
This nose is optimistic and outgoing—
you're enthusiastic and willingly work
for short-term goals. To make this nose
seem longer, make it appear narrower
—slightly darker foundation on each
side, a little highlight on the tip.

and this may apply to personal relationships, because you do not get too deeply involved; and when it comes to pairups, you often are the one who is chosen, not the one who makes the choice.

Cosmetically, there's really nothing wrong with your nose as it is. If you want it to look longer, your best approach is to make it look narrower. This gives apparent length. To do this, use a little slightly darker foundation on both sides of the nose—or a touch of taupe blusher—to make the sides narrower, and a little light foundation on the part of the nose between the nostrils and on the tip. If your nose looks longer, you will look more responsible—and its effect on your own psyche may be to make you feel more responsible, less devil-may-care about the future. In your forties, when characteristics related to the nose become most important, you might otherwise feel rather unsettled and missing out on the achievements that your contemporaries are enjoying. By way of compensation, your nose will always look young and eager and cheerful—and this attracts ever-new opportunities to look forward to.

5. Long Nose

This is the "thinker's nose," and if it is yours, you should go into one of the cerebral, mental professions where you can use your head— lawyer, writer, teacher, accountant, insurance, and so on. You are also capable of artistic achievement—but you tend to be conservative, as well as overrational, and often unrealistic, because you forget how much others are governed by their feelings and inner needs while you figure things out rationally and act intelligently in every case. You're a good helpmeet because you stay on a budget and understand its rationale, but you aren't a get-rich-quick person and prefer to build your assets gradually, and build for security rather than for instant gain. Your long nose give you a long-range view and you usually start young to plan for your old age.

If you want your nose to appear shorter, you can do it by making

LONG NOSE.
You are a thinker, an artist but not a get-rich-quick person. Build gradually for security rather than sudden gain. To make this nose seem shorter, make it appear wider by using makeup slightly paler than on the rest of the face, a little dark foundation under *the tip, peach blusher* on *the tip.*

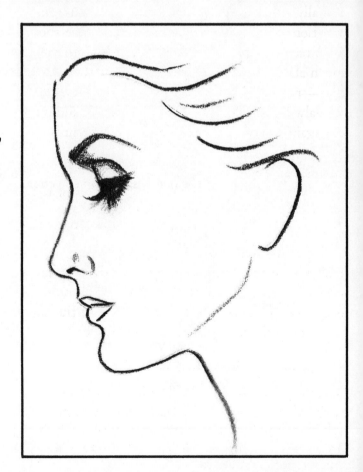

it appear wider. Do this by making the whole nose slightly lighter than the rest of the face, with a little dark foundation under the tip of the nose and a bit of peachy blusher on the tip.

As your nose tends to make you conservative, you will probably be very adverse to changes that may take place around you in your forties. Develop your creative and intellectual interests early so that you have many fields to fall back on when you reach these critical years.

6. Upturned Nose

The uptilted nose is youthful, attractive—and there is no reason usually to do anything to change it. It shows you to be cheerful, unconventional, and a free spender—generally a lighthearted upbeat person who doesn't worry about the future but unfortunately often wastes today. You're very generous with money—and may be overgenerous sexually, and as you cannot keep a secret, this can get you into ticklish situations. Many of the characteristics of the short nose apply to you —so read that section too. Actually, though you may not think too much about success, you *feel* successful always because the tip of the nose—the peak of perfection—is so well-developed. You are a person who always bounces back from any setback and is resouceful in starting out again when you are put down. This optimism is very attractive, so you have no trouble finding others to share your efforts and enthusiasms.

In your forties, when the characteristics of the nose become most prominent in life, you will probably still be starting out on new ventures and get happy results from whatever you try.

If you want to modify the uptilt of your nose, follow the instructions for the short nose, making it narrower by putting darker foundation on the sides, except that the nostrils need to be deemphasized even more with dark blusher and the tip of the nose should be covered over a broader area with peach-tone blusher.

7. Round-Tip Nose

This is the nose for money—which may surprise you. It's true. People with this shape nose accumulate wealth and thus are very good to have around in business or in the home. No, you won't be forever into deals —not an entrepreneur or get-rich-quicker. But you do accumulate

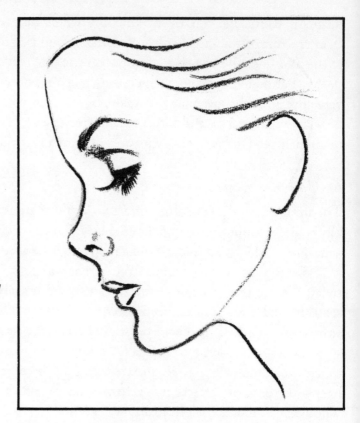

UPTURNED NOSE.
You are usually an upbeat light-hearted person—a free spender, and you cannot keep a secret. Narrow flaring nostrils with dark blusher, diminish the tip of the nose with peach-tone blush.

wealth and that's wonderful. The reason this will surprise you—and probably other people who know you—is that basically a round-tip-nose person is very kind hearted, warm, gentle spirited and self-sacrific-ing. You are in fact, a wonderful friend, an ideal wife and mother —the member of the family who helps out with sympathy and, if needed, cash to tide over the unfortunate relatives. You may not care about a career and certainly don't naturally seek venture capital and go into risky enterprises. Still, you get rich, because the nose represents Saturn, whose element is earth, and your nice round-trip nose accumu-lates and holds material things. You always end up financially secure —even well off—and this is true even if your main objective in life is completely different. Life in a sense rewards you for being such a good and kindly person—and you deserve a happy prosperous Peak of Per-fection (Point 48). Most employers will think of you as a hard worker and someone who will benefit the corporation—but they are not likely to recognize what a little gold mine you are. There's no reason to try

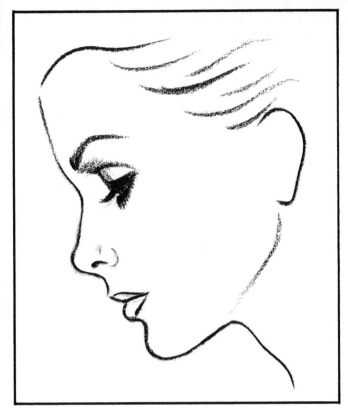

ROUND-TIP NOSE.
This is the nose for money—you end up well off, financially secure. Warm the tip with a slight peach blush or more color if it is pale or, if it is too rosy, tone down the color with foundation.

to change this bountiful nose. You come off as a nice person and you have, besides, inner beauty. You may only want to warm it up with a slight blush or more color if it is pale, to tone it down a little with color if it is too rosy (round noses often turn pink in the cold).

If you're asking yourself right now where all that money is, hang in. By the time you reach your forties, when the characteristics of the nose are shown most strongly, you will be financially secure—and finding new ways to make money all around you.

NOSTRIL TYPES

There are four types of nostrils that are important to the complete character of the nose. We are speaking now of the openings in the nose, not the outer flare of flesh that surrounds them. Look down into a mirror and see whether yours are square, triangular, round, or oval in their basic shape.

- Square nostrils indicate someone who is sturdy, reliable and likely to stick with any project to the bitter end.

- Triangular nostrils show stinginess, someone who is very careful and can even be mean about money (and perhaps also stingy about sex).

- Round nostrils show expediency, inventiveness and the capacity for finding original solutions to problems.

- Oval nostrils belong to the adventurer, one open to change and innovation.

Another point—nostril openings should be concealed, not visible when you look at your face straight on. Visible nostrils show a lack of modesty and tact.

The flare of the nostrils also modifies the shape of the nose and can somewhat change the fortune that your nose brings you.

- If the nostril flare is well proportioned and in balance with the size of the nose, it is helpful to any success the nose promises.

- If the nostril flares are large in proportion to the nose, they indicate a tendency to lose the money your nose has helped you accumulate, but if they are wide and flaring, you may become a self-made millionaire.

- Small narrow nostril flares in proportion to the size of the nose suggest caution in moneymaking; you will probably prefer to work for another and pocket a regular salary rather than taking chances on your own.

- If your nostrils are very thin and flat, you may have trouble both making money and hanging on to it.

Unfortunately, makeup can do little to change the flare of your nostrils, but skillful use of the face-balancing techniques (see chapter 7) and of making up the other features of the face, can minimize any disparity in the flare of the nostrils. If nostril flares are too large, minimize them with some dark foundation; if they are miniscule, enlarge their appearance with light foundation (as with a small nose). Rather than fussing around with this kind of "stage" makeup, however, it is best to make up the features you can change—the eyes, brows, and mouth—and let the nose and nostrils find their own proportion to the face.

COLOR

The color of the nose is important to its influence on your fortune. The nose represents Saturn, and Saturn is an earth planet. Its element is the soil and its color is beigy pink or *peach*. When you use a blusher to modify the shape and size of your nose, use it in a peachy shade or an amber shade if the skin is dark. This pinky-gold color promises good fortune in money matters and will naturally attract others who are able to help you make your fortune—you'll be a winner. A red nose does *not* indicate good health—or wealth—but rather loss, so don't risk your money with a red-nose partner. Grayish color on the nose indicates ailments; greenish, a default (you may even be jailed). But purplish color on the nose promises a promotion.

Interestingly enough, a shiny nose—the cosmetic catastrophe so long fought by the powder puff—is considered positive in Chinese Face Reading. It suggests prosperity and high favors and position. So don't freak out in a job interview or other business meeting if you feel your nose sweating or getting a glow. It will only indicate that you are headed for high honors.

Another thing not to worry about are freckles on your nose. In the Chinese art of Face Reading they're considered *sexy*.

The Mouth—Personality

ALONG WITH THE EYES, the mouth is the key to expression in the face. The mouth represents the *personality*—and also sensuality. So lipstick, rather than eye makeup, is naturally a young girl's first cosmetic, her first step toward sexual expression. The mouth serves not only for our being fed, but is also our instrument of expression in speech and is the medium of the kiss. No wonder we spend so much effort in making our mouth beautiful.

Oddly perhaps at first thought, the Position Points surrounding the mouth are not those of youth but the early fifties, with the mouth itself Position Point 60 and Position Point 70 underlying the lower lip. Not so surprising, though, when you consider that the Third Station, the lower part of the face, is that emphasized in old age and indicates longevity. The Palace of the Household also occupies the mouth area and this part of the face becomes more important in later life—your mouth, chin and jawline determine, along with how you live in early life, the quality and maintenance of life as you age.

Two Minor Features—the laugh lines (Positions 56 and 57) which represent longevity and run around the mouth from the flare of nostrils and operate when we smile, and the philtrum, the groove from the nostrils to the bow of the mouth (Position Point 51)—are near the mouth and relate to it.

The philtrum represents sexuality—fertility. And it is at age fifty that one may enjoy even more the results of one's fertility. One's children are producing grandchildren—and the individual has the pleasure of seeing her life force spread out and productive. The early fifties are also for some couples the time of the second honeymoon— when, free of the responsibilities of children, they discover each other again. For others, it is the "second adolescence" when new experiences, new loves, new adventures create a new life.

Position Point 60 in the middle of the mouth is the Point of Mercury—which represents water. Healthy lips are moist and rosy red with Mercury's color. The area under the lower lip (surrounding Point 61) is called the "sea of wine" and is a "travel" point. Full and lush, it enables you to travel far and wide.

The mouth, of course, is important to you all your life—from the moment you are born. And it's the face's bright beauty spot.

A good firm mobile mouth indicates a person of integrity, fine health, and pleasing personality. The lips should be fairly full, firm, and well shaped.

The mouth should be full and rounded, with both the upper and lower lip of equal fullness and the indentation in the upper lip well-defined. The corners of upper and lower lip should meet exactly.

Of course everyone can't have an ideal mouth—or should try to make hers over too much. Better to understand what your mouth means to your fortune and make it up to be most effective and then live with it.

What you want is the perfect mouth for you—the mouth that best expresses *your* personality and the aspect of your personality you want to emphasize for a special occasion. For example, if you are applying for a job in a stolid business firm, you will want your mouth to look smooth and balanced and confident. If you are out for fun, you may want it to appear luscious and appealing. If you are seeking new friends, you may want it to appear winsome and sweet. You can set the mood of your own mouth, whatever its shape or size, by the way you make it up and the colors you choose.

Ideally, the mouth should be made up to look moist and sensuous, but in today's business world, it is sometimes wise to play this down. Matte (no shine) makeup is considered more appropriate.

You can use a lipliner pencil or brush to improve the mouth's shape, but the main purpose of a lipliner is to give the mouth a definite outline. Rather than changing its outline by the use of a lipliner, it is better to use *color* to emphasize or modify the shape of the mouth. Bright and light color makes a part of the mouth stand out, darker color makes it more dramatic.

Usually a lipliner should be in a shade slightly darker than the lipstick or gloss you will be using. If you are using a ginger or brownish shade of lip color, you can even use a medium-brown brow pencil to line the lips. The line is there chiefly to give the mouth shape depth and contour, and should be covered by the lipstick or lip gloss. Lipliner also helps keep the color from spreading out onto the surrounding skin area.

Line the lips with either a pencil or brush. Start in the middle of the upper lip and work outward to each side; then start in the middle of the lower lip and work outward to the corners. Keep the line very fine in the corners of the mouth.

To line the lips well, rest your elbow on a table and rest the heel of your hand against your chin and your little finger against the cheek for support and work with small smooth strokes. Lip lining takes practice, but you can master it if you are patient. Follow the natural line of the flesh surrounding the lips, keeping the color within the natural line of the lips, not outside it. The lips should be relaxed, the mouth slightly open as you work. A pencil gives a smoother line; the brush a softer line; you may want to line the upper lip with a pencil, the lower with a brush.

You get a fuller, softer, more luscious look if you also fill in the color with a lipstick brush. Again, keep the lips relaxed and work in soft smooth strokes, filling in the upper lip first and then the lower lip.

If you want a matte look, dust some translucent powder over your lips when you have finished; it is quickly absorbed and gives a soft smooth look. If you want shine, use gloss only in the middle of the mouth. The very young may want to use only colored gloss for a shiny-mouth look.

DESIGNING YOUR MOUTH

The mouth represents the personality and also sensuality—and you are the one who knows what part of your personality you want to emphasize in your mouth makeup, what part you want to subdue. Here are some of the mouth patterns that indicate important personality traits and how to overcome any problems.

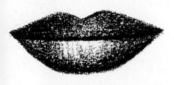

THE BALANCED MOUTH.
Keep lips of the same fullness and be sure corners meet exactly. Brighter color on the lower lip brings the whole mouth alive. This mouth shows an even temperament, openly friendly.

1. Balanced Mouth

The lips are of the same fullness and the corners meet exactly. Line and fill this mouth with precision and you should have no problems. Use a slightly brighter or lighter color on the lower lip so the whole mouth comes alive and catches the light. If this is your mouth, it reveals you as a person of warmth and charm, a responsible person in society and with the promise of great achievement in life. You probably express yourself naturally and easily, are pleasant to be with. You have an even temperament, are openly friendly, smile a lot, and enjoy spontaneous laughter. Your mouth shows good health and vitality, and a responsive sexual nature, with perhaps a tendency to want to share experiences on an equal basis without being either dominant or dependent. This mouth makes you a very equable handler of people, and you can succeed in work where you will have subordinates—and also work well for others if that is required of you.

In an executive position you may develop strong laugh lines at an earlier age than others—but you cope well with tension and are an easy acceptor of the pleasures and panics of social and business life. You are not one to go under in a tough situation and you adjust readily to changes. When you reach maturity, you will probably consider yourself happy and be very well satisfied with the environment you have made for yourself and your family.

You can deal with the public and are a fine spokeswoman for any organization that may make you its advocate. If the philtrum promises you children and grandchildren, you will be a respected and enjoyed parent and grandparent and are likely, because you are so congenial, to have created a happy, lasting marriage.

Because you are likely to be successful in a career, you may tend to make up your mouth too firmly and precisely as you get older; you have an orderly, even mind and will take on responsibilities. Remember that a mouth should be soft and delicate and inviting.

2. Crescent Mouth

This mouth turns up at the corners and usually has a well defined indentation on the upper lip—especially if the philtrum is deep. It shows you to be cheerful, optimistic, attractive, active, creative, liked by others. You have a delightful sense of humor and are always first to see the joke in any situation. You laugh a lot, and tend to smile—even at adversity. Your children find you a fun mamma, and your mate and you share good times and probably are very sociable. You are sensitive too and can ripple at times between tears and laughter, though the laughter usually quickly bubbles up. Your appearance of optimism and good humor helps you land jobs—if you have the aptitudes and skills to go with them—but because you're easygoing you may get bogged down with a humdrum kind of work. Don't. You need creativity—a chance to express your slightly offbeat insights. Try cartooning as a hobby—it may lead to the big time and big money. You would also be good at writing and drawing children's books, and if other things are substantiating, design, popular music—lyrics and melody—could be personal fulfillments. Whatever you do, you put a light touch into it that others appreciate and enjoy. You're a wonderful greeter—because you have a built-in smile, and work

CRESCENT MOUTH. Pencil the lower lip all the way to the corners to emphasize the uptilt, fill upper lip to full width and gloss upper and lower lip. This is a cheerful mouth—youthful and creative.

well in public relations. Luckily, you attract happy-go-lucky people, like yourself, and are never bored, though you are sometimes restless.

Because this is a naturally pleasing mouth, emphasize it. Pencil the lower lip all the way to the corners to emphasize the uptilt. If the upper lip is thinner than the lower lip, fill the outline of the upper lip to the full width and use gloss on the upper lip to give it strength. Using gloss only on the middle of the lower lip modifies the uptilt— as you may want to do sometimes in your more pensive moods.

This is a fortunate mouth for the later years because it always looks youthful and happy—and as this draws others to you, it can help keep you a lifelong cheerful person.

3. Bow-Shaped Mouth

This mouth tends to have a pouty look. Lower and upper lip are full and rounded but the corners are on much the same level as the curve of the lower lip. With this kind of mouth you may pride yourself on your cynicism, your rather dim view of everything, but others may read this as a lack of sensuality and find you too impersonal, rather self-centered. Actually, this is a tempting mouth, but you tend, because of your lack of faith in others, not to want to yield too much of yourself. Instead, you may become too self-indulgent and seek pleasure from food rather than from people. You tend to isolate yourself, not physically, because you do seek sociability and want others around you, but somehow keep aloof in a crowd and may even seem to look down on others somewhat. You are an ideal person to work in a place where many men will try to date you for business advantages, because you both tempt them and are able to see through their wiles and stand them off. You can do well in modeling and some aspects of show business because you are often playing a part. Once you are able to break down your defenses and feel that you can be trusting—that others aren't really just out to get everything they can—you can be sensual, warm and giving. Unfortunately, your very cynicism tends to attract the wrong kind of experiences for that. Try to be affectionate if you can't be sensuous, and find one person in whom you can place your confidence. If you don't, you may fall into promiscuous relationships, with none very meaningful.

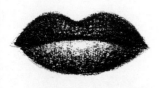

BOW-SHAPED MOUTH.
Pencil for a definite shape, sharpening the line of the upper lip and giving the lower lip full contour. Gloss all over to make the mouth seem wider. This is an impersonal cynical mouth—but sensual too.

In making up this mouth, use a pencil to give it a more definite shape—sharpening the line of the upper lip and drawing the line of the lower lip at a full contour, making sure that the lower corners are fuller. Use gloss all over the mouth to make it seem wider, more assured.

As the mouth tends to widen in the middle years, you may find yourself taking a broader view of life as you mature and become more positive as a result. As relationships at this time of life are often more objective, less personal, you may find more in common with both your contemporaries and the young—and become in effect a kind of "wise woman" to the younger generation.

4. Thin, Wide Mouth

This generous mouth with thin lips and a broad smile shows you to be proud, strongminded, authoritative and firm in decisions. True, others may find you too rigid, but you usually wear them down after a while as you have the type of personality that wins out. You're very energetic and generous and if you seem always to take charge, it's because someone has to, and you do it without creating rancor or resentment. You don't change your mind once you've made your decisions—and even if you can see the wisdom of it, you often don't feel it's worth the effort to start all over. You'd rather go on to other things that demand your authority. Your children will be well brought up and kept in line—but they will appreciate and really love you, just because you're so strong minded and aren't afraid to discipline them and really "know best." You and your mate may not always see eye to eye, but he will probably have the good sense to follow your judgment and feel you're right, which you usually are. This doesn't mean he's weak and you're domineering, just that you probably choose someone as adaptable and easygoing as you are rigid. And in a showdown you always back each other up.

With this mouth you make a good supervisor and will quickly rise, wherever you start, to a managerial position. Oddly enough, even in a position of authority, you prefer a feminine role—and even if not supersensual you are basically loving and respected.

You must avoid the habit of tightening your mouth—learn to keep your lips relaxed. As you smile easily, this should not be diffi-

THIN WIDE MOUTH. Draw the outline just outside the natural lip line—but very delicately and never all the way into the corners. Fill with lipstick; use lots of gloss so lips seem fuller. This mouth shows one who is energetic and generous and wants to take charge.

cult. A thin mouth with the lips relaxed and slightly parted looks less thin.

In makeup, draw the lipline just outside the natural lip line—but very carefully—and never all the way into the corners. Fill in with lipstick and then add lots of gloss so the lips appear fuller.

As this mouth, like all mouths, tends to get wider with age, you become more broadminded and cheerful in the middle years, and are not afraid to exercise your authority a bit. One thing—you are a talker as well as a doer, and become even more so as life goes on. Train yourself to be a listener, too, and don't insist on the last word (as you are likely to do right up to your own last words).

5. Small Mouth

If your mouth is miniscule, your vitality may be low and your health delicate, and this can keep you out of many activities. Take care that it does not also make you small-minded through lack of communication. Whether you marry and have children or work in a busy place, you still tend to be a loner and like to dwell on your own inner life more than to participate in that around you. That's too bad, because you often have a very neat view of things that others would appreciate. And if they think you want to be alone, they will leave you alone. Luckily, you'll probably always find another who wants to be alone and you can be alone together—sharing your inner thoughts and your often critical opinions of others. Whether single or part of a couple or even of a family, you probably most easily get involved with people through a common interest—a hobby, or pets, or music or books, or through the common ground of your career or profession. On the negative side, you often lack the vitality it takes to keep up with others and often drop out. Really great opportunities are lost just because you can't make the effort.

A small mouth needs a lot of brightening for its psychological effect on you as well as for its invitation (which a mouth should be) to others to get interested in you.

Outline your lips all the way to the corners. Use lots of gloss on both the upper and lower lip to brighten the look and catch the eye. If the groove on your upper lip is deep, you really have a great deal of unexpended sensuality and will be happier if you indulge your really deep passions.

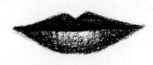

SMALL MOUTH. Outline lips all the way to the corner. Use lots of gloss on both lips for an illusion of size. This mouth shows delicacy, one who is a loner and has a rich inner life but may be hypercritical.

If your mouth is small to start with, avoid the habit of pursing your lips because this can give you a pinched look and detract from your attractiveness, especially as you reach the fifties, when the importance of the personality is emphasized. The main problem with your small mouth is that your whole personality can become encapsulated while you are young and never expand to its full radiance and expression.

6. Fish Mouth

The corners of your mouth droop and you often tend to keep your mouth slightly open, which emphasizes the effect. This mouth may appear innocent, but it actually shows one who is strong-willed and demanding, not easily influenced by others, and even tending to be domineering. You are quite capable of fighting for your rights—and will. A great many women have this shape of mouth and are thought to be gullible, but their would-be swindlers soon discover who in fact was taken in. No one with this mouth should be taken to be one of the weaker sex—it's a very useful mouth in a society that still expects women to be dependent and then demands of them a great deal of strength in dealing with everyday problems. In a sense, it's a fun mouth, because you tend to be sensual and to enjoy being lazy. Usually, you can nag or push others to going out and getting what you want and doing what you want done. You don't really want to do things for yourself—but pressed into it, you can and do.

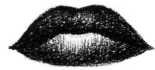

FISH MOUTH.
Line lips to cut the sides of the upper lip but do not carry the line all the way into the corners. Give the lower lip complete fullness and a slight lift at the outer tip. Gloss the middle of the lower lip only. This mouth is strong-willed and demanding.

In your work, you may not want to be at the top and have too much responsibility, but you do like to be in a position where you can make demands on others and order them about, and when you are so placed you usually get results. The problem with the droopy mouth is that it tends to look depressed and so makes the owner look overserious about everything. It also reveals too clearly the demanding nature that lies behind it.

Line your lips to cut the sides of the upper lip, but do not carry the line all the way to the corner. The lower lip needs filling out to be strengthened, and the corners brought up. Carry the line of the lower lip all the way to the corners and even give a slight lift at the outer tip. Use gloss only on the middle of the lower lip.

As the corners of this mouth tend to droop even more as you grow older, you have to guard against looking depressed and feeling depressed as you reach your early fifties, when there is strong emphasis on personality. Take care not to press people out of your life as you go along, because you will need their support and kindness later. Your natural sensuality will increase as you get older, and you need others with which it can find expression.

7. Cherry Mouth

If this full, round mouth—shaped like a kiss—is yours, you are gentle, kind, and quiet in nature and have very easy, tender, warm relationships. In fact, you are the ideal wife and probably before you've had time to think twice, some fine stalwart male has husbanded you. With this mouth a woman tends to marry young and to be very very happy. No woman with this mouth ever finds the housewife state or marriage restrictive. There are many people of all ages who seek you out, many things to do, many activities from arts and crafts to creative music, poetry, architecture, medicine, law, or whatever to call to you—and with any career you choose, you still are the perfect wife. You are imaginative, poetic, and practical; you are a gentle, loving mother and very easy to work with at any level. You are also a perfect hostess, and know the right thing to say and say it graciously.

Because it's so much in your nature to please, others may think you are merely docile and obedient. Actually, your cheerful and loving nature is usually very happily expressed in life, and in your early fifties, when your personality is at its fullest development, you are usually appreciated as someone of many gifts, and have found good fortune as a consequence.

Shape your mouth carefully with a pencil to bring out its full roundness and classical outline. Use lip gloss all over to emphasize its pretty shape.

CHERRY MOUTH.
Shape the mouth carefully with a pencil to bring out its full roundness and fullness. Gloss all over to emphasize its pretty shape. This mouth is gentle, creative—the sign of the perfect wife.

CHOOSING YOUR LIPSTICK COLORS

Lip colors are fashion colors—they should coordinate with the clothes you wear. They have very little to do with complexion color—except that you might perhaps, if very fair, choose from the lighter range of colors, and if very dark, from the deeper range. There is no reason today to have problems from complexion color because your foundation shade can always make your skin warmer if you are pale or sallow, and you can always add more blush; or if your skin is florid you can cool the redness with more beigy tones of foundation and blusher.

Lip colors are promoted each season to coordinate with the clothes colors that are being offered, and with the general trend in fashion as it swings to neutrals, to brights, or to pale colors. For this reason, it is important not to date yourself by using the same lip color year in and year out. Change with the fashion.

You may have a variety of clothes colors in your wardrobe, but you will find that they basically come down to three groups—the warm colors, those in the yellow to warm brown range; the cool colors, blues and greens, from light to dark; and the neutrals, grays, beiges, black, neutral browns.

Lipsticks fall into the same three categories:

- Warm—coral, peach range, orange
- Cool—rosy pinks
- Neutrals—ginger, beige, browns

If you pick a neutral shade, you can probably wear it with any of the three groups, but you will probably want a cool shade for wear with lilacs, pinks, blues, and other pastels in spring and summer, and a warm color if you wear lots of orange, warm browns, yellows, and ginger browns, especially in fall. For daytime you would perhaps choose a neutral that is not too bright. For evening, a more intense, deeper or shimmering lip color.

Lipsticks also range in shades from the lightest through the medium range to the deeper tones.

- The lightest, especially in the neutrals, give little color, and are often chosen by the very fair skinned and the youngest group, who want a very natural look.

- The medium range is most useful. Not too light or too dark, so that most women can wear them.

- The deeper tones are worn by those who have a very dark com-

plexion or by others for evening because they give a more sophisticated look.

Most women can get along well with three lip colors—a neutral in a
medium shade for day, a warm or cool shade to go with their wardrobe's dominant color, and a more intense shade (warm, cool, or
neutral) for evening.

As the fashion look of the mouth varies from pastel to bright to
neutral to deep, it's a good idea when you buy a new lipstick to intro-
duce a new fashion shade rather than replacing an old standby.

Very young girls often prefer lip gloss in a transparent color to a
lipstick. It gives shine with a minimum of color.

Avoid colors that are too bright, too garish, too bizarre.

The younger woman needs slightly brighter colors, and will find
the earth colors (neutrals) beautiful with a tan.

The more mature require a slightly deeper color to perk up the
face—but not overly bright. Mature women should carefully line
their lips because it prevents the lip color's bleeding into any tiny
lines around the mouth. (Another way to avoid this bleeding is to
powder the skin around the lips.) When you line your lips, do not
use a dark pencil, as this becomes too dramatic. Instead, pencil the
lips with a light color and keep the line within the lipline, and cover
it with your lipstick. If lips are somewhat crinkly, use a soft pastel
color to make this wrinkling less noticeable.

TEETH

Although the teeth aren't one of the Five Major or Seven Minor
Features of the face, they still are vital to good looks and have significance in the Chinese art of Face Reading.

- If your teeth are white, straight, of medium size and tightly placed,
  they promise intelligence, character and well-being, and speak of a
  person who is very much together.

- Rounded teeth, nicely fitted together and very white are super-
  special. They show you to be artistic, intelligent, gifted in many
  ways—a very harmonious and interesting person.

- If teeth are very long, they promise a long life, but you will have to work hard for anything you want. Life will not be gentle, and nothing will come easily.

- If teeth slant inward, you are likely to be lonely—or like to be alone.

- If teeth are crooked, their owner is not to be trusted; the personality is said to be devious—frankly "crooked" (a good reason for teeth-straightening!).

- Very small teeth with a lot of gum showing indicates a very selfish individual who will have only his or her own interests at heart; this indicates someone to watch out for, and not become too intimate with.

- Space between the two front teeth indicates that the owner will be unhappy in her old age—not socially well off—and will develop family problems.

- The left front top tooth indicates loyalty to country and to society; the right front top tooth indicates filial piety—relationship to parents. If one is crooked, it shows a deviation in loyalties either to family or the state.

As far as the natural color of teeth is concerned, though white is cosmetically ideal, some teeth are naturally shaded toward yellow or toward blue. If teeth have natural yellow tones, coral or orange tones in lip colors or brown or ginger neutrals will make them look whiter; if teeth tend toward blue, a cool lip color will make them appear whiter.

Luckily, today something can be done about most kinds of teeth. Tooth straightening, capping, and now "tooth painting" (a means of correcting discoloration, correcting small chips, and even rebuilding a broken tooth without grinding it down for capping) and small removable devices to slip over the front teeth to hide a "gap" are available. A good dentist is indeed a girl's best friend.

And of course, keeping your teeth in good shape is one of the best defenses against the marks of premature age—deep lines around the mouth, hollow cheeks, thinning of the lips. Getting any missing teeth replaced, practicing good nutrition to preserve the jawbone, and attention to gum problems can help preserve your tooth beauty—and maybe avoid cosmetic surgery.

As the Position Points 51–55 and 70 cluster around the mouth and the mouth itself is Point 60, these are the years when good teeth can help your looks, vitality and personality considerably.

Will correcting your dental problems change your fate? Not as far as the inborn traits go—but as far as your attitude toward yourself is concerned and the impression you make on others, it can indeed.

The Ears—Potential

THE EARS are one of the Five Major Features and, according to Chinese Face Reading, tell much about your potential in life. Cosmetically, though, there is little you can do for them—except cover them with your hair, have them surgically "pinned back" if they protrude, or emphasize them with earrings. Their importance to the overall appearance of your face—and to your approach to life—makes them worth thinking about. Besides, you can learn a great deal about others by looking at their ears, and because the male often has his ears showing, their characteristics are a big help in picking a life partner.

Position Points 1 to 7 are on the left ear—and represent the influence of the father and also of the planet Jupiter. Position Points 8 to 14 are on the right ear and represent the influence of the mother and of the planet Venus.

The ear is said to resemble in form the fetus in the womb—and today's medical researchers back up its significance by relating defects in the form of the ear to prenatal brain malformations and even predict heart attack by a line that forms in the lobe in later life. Well-shaped ears indicate a happy childhood, prosperity, long life, and fine children.

Although the early years (through age thirteen) are indicated by the Position Points on the ears, the ears themselves are located in the

Second or middle Station of the face, which controls early maturity—the period when you do most to create your own success. The relationship is clear, because the start you get in early life and the influence of your parents bear strongly upon this part of your life and your ability to make a success of your work, as well as to meet the responsibilities of being a parent yourself.

The positioning of the ears on the head relates closely to what you will do for yourself in life:

- If the ears are set high, so that the top of the ear is higher than the top of the eyebrows, you are an unusual person—an early achiever and superintelligent.

- If the tops of the ears rise only to the space between the tip of the brow and the corner of the eye, you are among the most successful in life. You are more likely to do well in business and carry the burden of responsibility. You are destined for a kind of high position and rely on your own initiative to make your place in the world.

- If your ears are low set, so the tip of the ear is at the level of the outer tip of the eye or lower, you achieve late in life. Often you are perfectly happy to let others work for you and little inclined to do things for yourself. If a man's ears are set this low, he often will let his wife support him. If a woman's ears are low, she is happy to be dependent on her mate and won't be making much effort on her own behalf.

- The ears should be set close to the head, but not too tight. People with protruding ears are considered easygoing, but the owners may easily lose things and may be irresponsible. Such ears also signify sexual promiscuity.

The size of the ears has significance too—large, long ears, if well formed, are considered desirable. Large, poorly shaped ears, though, are a liability and reflect a disorganized nature. Very small ears, particularly if not well formed, can mean limitations.

The ear is divided into three parts:

- The outer rim should be well formed and moderately fleshed for longevity and good health and achievement; if it is thin, it shows a lack of sexual vitality.

- The inner rim indicates emotions. If it protrudes outward, you are a good mixer; if it turns inward, you tend to be reclusive and to repress your feelings.

- The third and most significant part of the ear is the lobe. In Chinese Face Reading it is called the "Pearl Drop." It should be pale pink and have the delicate rounded sensitivity of a pearl. It is of course also the place where we wear pearl drops—our earrings.

The Position Points of the lobe are numbers 5, 6, 7 on the left ear, representing the end of early childhood; and numbers 12, 13, 14 on the right ear, which represents the end of puberty and the beginning of adolescence—the first year of the teens (age thirteen). Very long, the lobe represents vitality and longevity; firm and rounded, prosperity and a good life.

EAR PIERCING AND SURGERY

Many of the nerves connected with the brain and body have centers in the lobe of the ear. And this raises one of the most important cosmetic points about the ear—ear piercing.

If you have your ears pierced, you should wait till you are well into your teens and even then have the piercing done very carefully and by a professional. Prematurely or carelessly placed ear holes can be damaging to the nerves of the lobe and can lead to problems later in life. As you have probably heard, the so-called "acupuncture diet" relies on a staple being put in the ear at a particular point to control appetite. This relates to the nerve (or acupuncture lines) connected to the digestive tract. We have also mentioned the transverse line that appears at the top outer edge of the lobe that is a warning of possible heart attack in middle age. This all goes to show the sensitive nature of the lobe and its relationship to health, and indicates why caution in ear-piercing is necessary.

Surgery to reduce floppy ears is often done as early as the age of seven—but it can be done at any time after that. Better later, because children sometimes grow into their ears and the floppiness is not as noticeable later. If it creates a psychological problem, it is certainly worth the rather simple surgical correction.

EAR TYPES

Here are seven major ear types and what they signify:

1. Large Ear

You may think of it as a defect—something to be covered by your hair—but think of it now as an asset. It signifies an alert, healthy individual—one with good character, a happy childhood, one who will enjoy a long fruitful life. If well placed, this is a good ear for business, even though women with large ears have a tendency to cover them

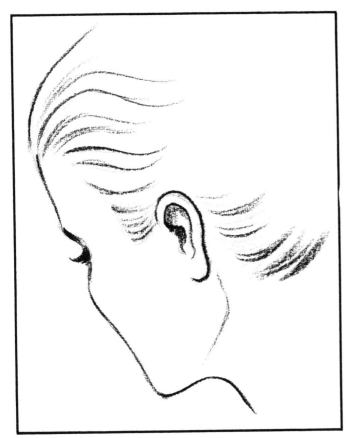

LARGE EAR.
Indicates good character, happy childhood, long fruitful life. Cover large ears with hair or modify them with tawny-rose blusher on the lobes.

altogether or at least partly with their hair. If you are a business-woman, don't be afraid to expose them—because others are sublim-inally impressed by large ears: they show acumen, vitality, and power. One of the great ladies of the cosmetic business had large ears, and she always exposed them, wearing her hair sleeked back into a bun. Of course, she also had other impressive business features—her nose, eyes, cheekbones, jaw—to support her ears. And large ears must always be considered in relation to the size of the rest of the face. If your large ears are too dominant, shadow them with hair, and modify them with medium (wedding-ring size) gold hoop earrings. A little tawny-rose blusher on the lobes will help them recede, though the color of the ears is preferably pinky-white and the ears preferably should be lighter than the face. In the case of large prominent ears, make an exception.

Just bear in mind that this ear promises you a rewarding life and that ears tend to lengthen as we get older. The long your lobe, the more wisdom and spirituality you will acquire as you get older.

2. Pointed Ear

If this is your ear, it shows that you are shrewd, capable of making a point in a business deal. But you must be wary of becoming a drifter in life, as you tend to ficklemindedness and often are too much of an opportunist, leaving destruction in your wake. People tend to distrust someone with pointed ears. In Greek mythology, they are associated with the mischief-making, fun-loving faun—half man, half goat—and in northern European folklore, with the changeling, the elf, who was substituted for the infant in the crib and was a constant source of trouble to the often unsuspecting parents. If you tend to have this kind of ear and to be this kind of wild child, look for other features on your face that will give you stability. You are better off not working in banks or as a business cashier or in other places where you are subject to temptation, because you tend to think of the present moment and not about future consequences of your actions. You will probably be impulsive in relationships, tend to shift jobs often, and be on the out-look for instant opportunities for a quick deal. Luckily, you are astute and can make brilliant deals when you are into a transaction—just try to keep on the right side of the law because you are not naturally averse to shady enterprises. Because you instill distrust in others, it is a good idea to keep your ear tips covered. The "faun" hairdo—often called the "Italian boy," "Greek fisherman," and other names to update it—with short curls that cover your pointy ears while still reflecting your active mercurial nature and innate charm, is a happy solution. If you encounter this ear in others, be careful of entrapment by their fast talk, and will-of-the-wisp schemes, but take advantage in business of their native astuteness, which can be helpful to less quick-thinking people. Those with this ear quickly "get the point" of any situation and know how to make the most of it quickly.

3. Round Top, No Lobe

With this ear you are idealistic and have a good family background, but your successes may be short lived, because the lobe is absent. En-

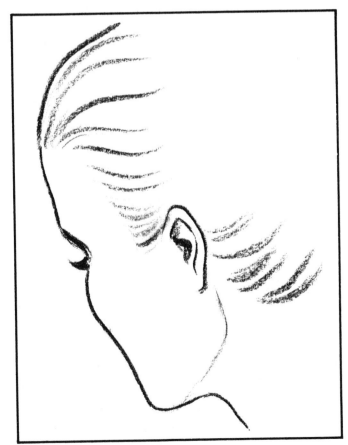

POINTED EAR.
Its owner is impulsive, an opportunist, but astute, has innate charm. Short curls that cover the points are helpful as many people distrust this ear.

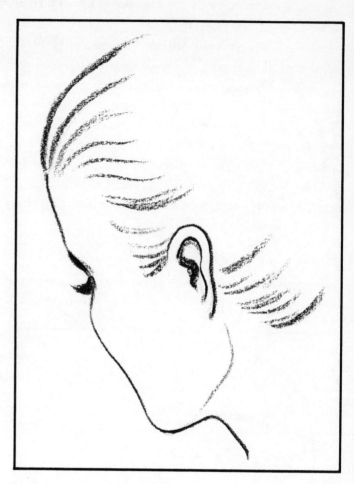

ROUND TOP, NO LOBE.
Its owner is idealistic, adaptable to
change. If well formed this ear offers no
beauty problems—except that it is
hard to wear earrings because the lobe
is absent.

joy the present and its advantages but don't rely too heavily on future plans. Luckily, with this ear you are easily adaptable to change and make adjustments in personal relationships and business ups and downs very lightly. You can be happy, too, with pleasant day-to-day experiences, and as a result, opportunities often drop in your lap. Unfortunately, with this ear you find it hard to wear earrings. Many models, fashion and beauty, have this ear—and are of course noted for their early and brief success, but they do have problems if they are asked to wear certain earrings for a fashion photo. You can wear the kind that circle the ear, or those that follow natural curve of the ear. Because this ear is usually small (it is shorter than other ears), if also well formed, it offers no beauty problem.

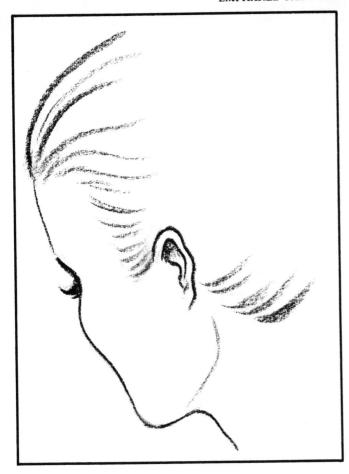

IRREGULAR EAR.
Impulsive, restless, tending to be
irresponsible, a drifter. Cover this ear
with your hair and wear a pendant
earring so that the ear appears longer
than it is.

4. Irregular, Small, with No Lobe

This is the ear of someone who has perhaps come from a broken home or otherwise was given a poor start in life. You tend to take chances, are impulsive and restless, moving often from place to place, and rarely form long relationships. You may prefer life as an irresponsible swinging single, because you tend to have a grasshopper mind and move quickly from one thing to another. If this is your ear, cover it with your hair and wear a pretty pendant earring so that the ear appears longer. As other features in your face probably compensate for your poor beginnings, you have to look elsewhere for the confidence and companionship that you may basically need. If you see this ear on another, you can spot him or her as an offbeat personality, likely to be a heartbreaker or a defaulter.

5. *Large Ear with Long Lobe*

This is an excellent ear. Your nature is spiritual, with high wisdom and nobility of character, and you can expect to live a very long life. As your success in life grows as you get older, you should not be too impatient in youth when you are developing your powers. With this ear you may tend to withdraw at times from the humdrum of the business world and take time out from pursuing a practical goal. But your values keep you in a fairly well oriented position as far as income and comfort go. Your physical needs may be relatively few compared with your intellectual and spiritual goals, and if you pursue your inner wisdom you will probably reach a high position as a spiritual leader, judge, or educator, or even in the healing professions. You can modify your long earlobe with a touch of tawny-pink blusher on the lobes. The color of the ears is naturally pinkish-white, but make an exception in your case. As the lobe of the ears gets longer as you age, and you are going to live a long, long time, don't stretch it with heavy earrings in your youth.

6. *Small Ear*

This is the sign of a stable, active self-made person who finds success in the middle years. As the small ear is usually well formed, you have no problems. Show it off by wearing off-the-ear hairdos when you choose, adorn it with pretty earrings. Others naturally admire and trust this ear. Depending on its setting—high, low, or medium—you will achieve much for yourself, or let others work for you, or be happy in a middle position. But you are usually extremely competent at whatever you choose to do, and have stable rewarding personal relationships that become warmer as you mature. You want to create your own environment, and as you probably have a keen sense of sound and color, you tend to live in beautiful surroundings with many comforts about you—and everything in exquisite taste. As you tend to be a conformist, you may in your later years be less adaptable than is necessary for you to cope with changes. Stable yourself, you seek stability in others and in your society. It is a good idea to form close attachments to a social group that supports—in a sense, guarantees—the persistence of your values, because changes will come hard, though once you make them, you are very contented.

7. Large Ear with Protruding Inner Rim

You are independent, successful, worldly, but basically a noncon-formist and thus may find it hard to establish your place in the ordi-nary business world. Look for a field where you can be your own woman—sales, advertising, the arts—and have a say in how things are going to be. You are likely to be very sociable and voice your views too ardently and be forever on the lookout for new people, new ex-periences. But basically, you are successful—and make your mark in whatever you attempt. A woman of the world, in the sense of being sophisticated and enjoying sophisticated company, you should look to cities for employment, because you need to have a chance to stretch your personality through contacts with others. People with this ear are often found far from their place of origin.

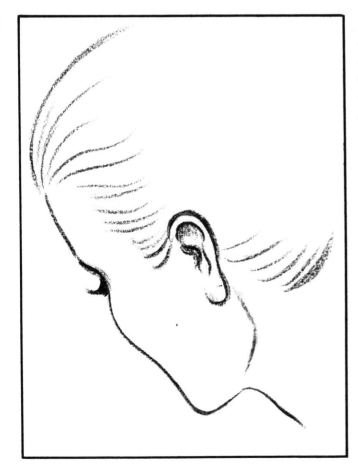

LARGE LONG LOBE.
High wisdom, noble character, long life—these are granted by a long-lobed ear. But expect success to come somewhat late in life. Button earrings modify the long lobe.

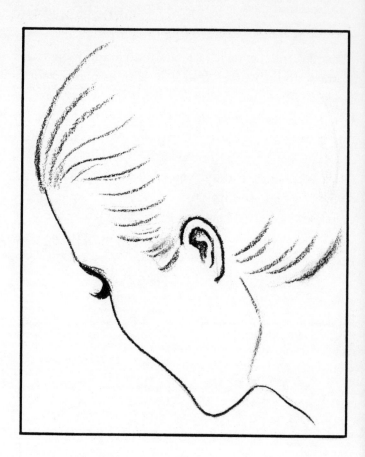

SMALL EAR.
A beauty asset—show off dainty ears
with off-the-ear hairdos, adorn with
pretty earrings. Others trust this ear
because it shows a stable, competent
individual.

You are so independent that you aren't going to care whether your ears seems too big, or look a little odd to others. You do what you choose and are likely to affect dramatic earrings and other offbeat accessories and to wear your hair in a dramatic style. You are very fashion-conscious and are always first or near first to display a new style, and you wear it exactly as it was meant to be worn—with flair. This is because your inner ear is quick to pick up changing trends and new concepts that are reflected in fashion. In fact, you do very well in the fashion and creative fields, and can become a leader—a trend-setter—rather than simply a follower.

EAR COLOR

Ideally, the color of the ears is pinkish white. The ears should be lighter than the face. Too red, they reflect ill health or an angry tem-

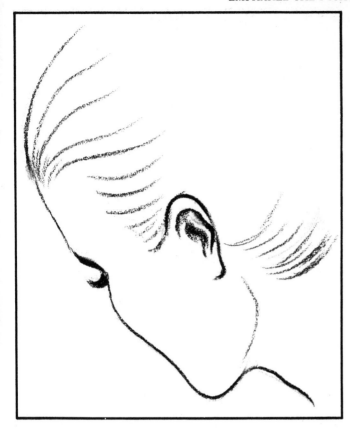

PROTRUDING INNER RIM.
This indicates a nonconformist—
independent, successful, worldly.
Emphasize this ear with dramatic
earrings and hair style.

perament. In general, it isn't necessary to make up your ears. If they are dark, too red, or too shiny, you may want to cover the outer rim with your foundation. The only other makeup trick with ears is to put some pink blush on the lobes in the evening. This gives brightness to the face, and diminishes the apparent size of the lobes if they are too long or large.

EARRINGS

Earrings are the "cosmetic of the ears." But actually, the shape of the earring relates more to the shape of the bottom part of the face—the chin and jaw—than to the ear itself. Long pendant earrings lengthen the jaw. Fat button earrings widen the jaw area. Hoop earrings modify a sharp chin. Small earrings simply call attention to a pretty ear and are a pleasant fashion touch.

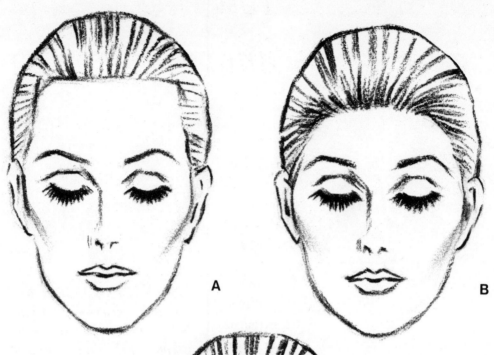

(A) HIGH AND SQUARE. *Intellectual ability, good family background and education, and excellent values.*

(B) LOW, ROUNDED. *Indicates a poor start in life, with a deprived childhood, difficulty in getting an education.*

(C) ROUNDED, NO ANGLES. *A harmonious individual, probably not aggressive or very ambitious; often reserved. Childhood usually pleasant but not stimulating.*

6. Pointing Up Your Good Points— The Seven Minor Features

MANY WOMEN, in making up their faces, emphasize a poor feature—such as bushy eyebrows—thinking it gives them character, and ignore or play down a good one (who needs a high forehead?). When you understand your own face—including the Seven Minor Features—you won't make such mistakes.

The Seven Minor Features are "minor" in that they form the framework and "fill" for your face and are a background for The Major Features. They indicate your inner drives, your strengths and weaknesses—the characteristics that constrain or compel you. They are, nevertheless, important both to your personality and your appearance.

The Seven Minor Features are:

- The forehead—indicating character.
- Cheekbones—showing power.
- Jawline—revealing life situation (status).
- Chin—demonstrating strength.
- Philtrum, the groove between lips and nose—life force, reproductive capacity, productivity. If deep, you are very sensual.
- Laugh lines—longevity.
- Undereye area—children, productivity.

The Forehead—Character

THE FOREHEAD shows your character. It occupies the entire First Station of Life—Position Points for the years of the teens and twenties appear in this part of the face. Several Palaces, including the Palace of Achievement, showing what kind of a start you get in life, are here. The Stage Coaches (Palaces of Transfer) which you observe for travel conditions are at the left and right of the upper tip of the brows. Between ages fourteen and thirty, the traits shown by the forehead are the most pervasive in your life.

FOREHEAD FEATURES

The forehead should be clear and well shaped and in balance with the rest of the face—about as long from the hairline to the brows as from the brows to the tip of the nose. The width of the forehead should be about the same as the width of the jaw. This creates a balanced face. The forehead should also be well-rounded, neither bulging or too flat.

High and Square

This shows good intellectual ability and excellent values, with fine family background and strong mental powers.

Low, Rounded

This indicates a possibly unpleasant or deprived childhood, with difficulty in getting an education. You probably did not get a good start in life and will have to develop other parts of the face to balance out your poor start.

Rounded, No Angles

This is a peaceable forehead, and its owner is probably not too aggressive or ambitious. You are often reserved; your childhood was probably pleasant, but you possibly were not stimulated enough.

Often people with low or rounded foreheads, though they get off to a bad start, are self-made because they have more power in the Second (middle) Station, where what one does with oneself comes into prominence.

Flat and Low

This means you will have to work hard in your youth for everything you get, with little help from your family.

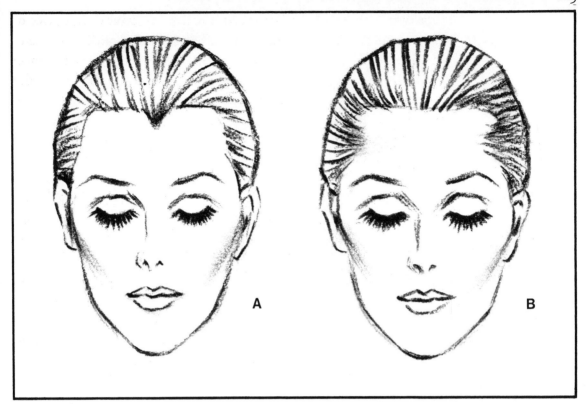

HAIRLINES

How the hair grows on the forehead is also significant to your character. If the hairline is uneven and the forehead is high, that's not troubling. If the forehead is low and the hairline is ragged, it indicates a more complex person.

If hair is coarse and bristly, an uneven hairline may be untidy in appearance. Models and actresses sometimes have such a hairline waxed so the line is clean. But only the barest fringe of tiny hairs along the hairline should be removed—just enough so that the hairline looks tidy but not unnatural. If fine, these tiny hairs along the hairline are not usually cosmetically troublesome, though in character they still show some early instability to overcome.

Hair that grows to a point in the middle of the forehead—called in the Western world a "widow's peak" because its owner was supposed to be destined to become a widow at an early age—is considered

(A) THE PEACH BLOSSOM.
A widow's peak indicates one who has charm and does well for herself, but is possibly self-centered.

(B) TEMPLE POINTS. Indicate one who is creative, artistic, alert, with a complex personality.

lucky in Chinese Face Reading. This peak in Chinese Face Reading is called the Peak of the Belle—indicating charm and flirtatiousness—or the Peach Blossom. A person with a Peach Blossom is romantic, has many affairs and is good in money matters—very much together, capable, adventurous, and creative, and does well for herself. True, a woman with a forehead peak may be self-centered but she always manages to take care of herself beautifully. This is Position Point 15—Mars—and is a Point of Strength. (Widowhood in Chinese Face Reading is indicated by high cheekbones, square jaw, and a bony bump on the nose.)

Hair that comes in at the temple to a point on each side of the forehead is also considered a blessing. Such a person is very creative, artistic and alert. And though the character may be complex, and perhaps hard for others to cope with and understand, it shows a person with vision and creative spirit.

If the hairline is strongly angular, it shows executive capacities and resourcefulness and its owner is strongly career oriented.

As it's unwise to try to do much about your hairline (except possibly to clean up its unevenness as mentioned above), the choice is really whether to make something of it by wearing your hair away from your face or to bring the hair forward and onto your face to modify your hairline.

Actually, because the forehead is the feature of youth and character and the current fashion is for a clear face, the forehead should be kept uncluttered in your teens and twenties to give yourself exposure and take advantage of the youthful look. Wear bangs only if you are a child under fourteen. Women in their thirties and forties should also keep their foreheads clear, again just because the look is youthful, and it gives a more open challenging face. If you are older and are bothered by forehead lines (see below), some fluff around your upper face may be softening.

If the forehead is very high and the hairline uneven, sideswept bangs, especially if the hair is straight and worn medium to long, break the height and still give you an open-face look. If hairline is uneven, short curls brought in at the sides and forehead from a surrounding mass of curls are also useful. Another solution is a geometric cut—especially good if the forehead is high and broad.

If the forehead is very low, the more the hair is brought away from it the better. Also keep the top hair rather flat—as volume in the hairdo will make the forehead seem smaller.

If hair grows in at a slant to narrow the forehead, it is wise to keep the hair pulled back from these wings, again to show all the forehead you can.

The forehead peak—Peach Blossom—is pretty and should be exposed by brushing hair back and away from it without a parting. A parting in the middle simply breaks up this attractive feature.

If the forehead is too rounded—bulging—and the hairline is also rounded, a side part with hair asymmetrical, cutting across part of the forehead, will be becoming.

Showing the forehead is especially important in young people looking for jobs or working in positions of authority, because it commands respect. But if the forehead is too high and bold, this may make you look overly "bossy," so you can well soften it.

The color of the forehead, which is ruled by Mars (fire) should be pinkish, so a light dusting of blusher in the middle can be used. If you have a high forehead, a light streak of pink blusher along the hairline can modify the apparent height.

The forehead should also glow. As this is a part of the face's natural "oil field" (like the nose, it has many oil and sweat glands), it will usually glow naturally, a sign of good health and good character —and *lucky*.

FOREHEAD LINES

Are you worried about forehead lines? Don't be. According to Chinese Face Reading, most of them are fortunate. There is little you can do about them—they are genetic in their formation—except that you should not exaggerate them by wrinkling your forehead (the transverse lines) or frowning (the vertical lines between the brows). Instead, count your lines and count your blessings.

If you have only one line and it is high, it can bring success. If it is low, it is not so fortunate. You will probably be limited in your accomplishments.

If you have two lines, it is very good. You have superintelligence, are a self-starter and an achiever.

If you have three lines, you don't have to be clever. This gives you a good position in life and nice things without having to work hard for them. Your life will be easy without much effort.

Also consider the Position Points at which the lines cross the forehead, or at which a line starts.

- Point 16 below the hairline is called Middle Sky and indicates the position in life of being the ruler, of being at the height or at the top of things.

- Point 19 is the Court of Heaven and indicates the position in life of being a cabinet minister or adviser to the ruler.

- Point 22 is the Steward of Heavenly Business—in which you are more or less running the show, possibly chancellor of the exchequer or office administrator.

- Point 25 is the Center of Heaven—a kind of center of pomp or display. If this point is shiny or emphasized you are very much in the public eye.

- Point 28, between the brows, is the Shrine of the Seal of Heaven where the mark of approval or acceptance is placed on you.

Between the brows, two vertical lines are normal—these two lines show a fine mentality and a great deal of cultural and intellectual prowess. More than three vertical lines here are not considered lucky. A person with more than three is likely to dissipate intellectual effort and scatter forces.

One line in this position is, however, a liability. This single line in Position 28 is called the "suspending needle" and indicates disappointment. A person with such a line may make a brilliant start, will be very creative and bright, but have a lot of disappointments. Writers, for example, often have this line. They have a lot of tension in going through life with a lot of pressure and a lot of disappointments.

Although the positions and number of these lines are from an early age indicated in the forehead and between the brows when you wrinkle your forehead or frown, they gradually become etched there only with use and time. Keeping your skin soft and supple makes them less noticeable, and if you protect your forehead skin against too much sun damage, use a moisturizer, and get any vision correction to avoid squinting, they can remain much modified till quite advanced years.

It is in youth, however, that the habit of wrinkling your forehead and frowning or squinting develops—and this is the time to become conscious of too much puckering up of the forehead and to guard against it. The same is true of oversunning. If you have a fair, sensitive skin, it is the damage done in your teens and twenties that shows up in wrinkles when you are in your forties and fifties. Suntan lotions that let you get a tan and yet protect the skin from harmful ultra-violet-B (burning) rays are available.

The Cheekbones—Power

LIKE THE NOSE, CHIN, AND FOREHEAD, the cheekbones are "mountains" of the face and should be prominent. The cheekbones show your power. Position Points 46 and 47 are on the points of the cheekbones, and the mid-forties is the age at which a whole generation begins to take over the power of a society in business, politics, education, communications, and the arts. It is usually the time when one achieves authority at the job and makes policies felt. If you are young and starting your career, those in the mid-forties will probably be your bosses. In the mid-forties the cheekbones actually become more prominent on the face as the bone structure begins to stand out.

The cheekbones not only show your power in career and public life, but they have to do with the quality of your marriage and your success as a mate. There is politics in family life as well as in national life, and a "balance of power" is needed for a successful relationship.

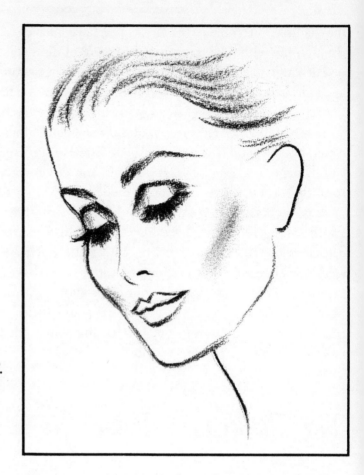

STRONG BASE, STRONG BONE.
Shows good background, prestige and
power, but perhaps someone who is
hard for others to get along with.

Luckily, there is a lot you can do with makeup to strengthen or modify the cheekbones, and to emphasize or deemphasize your impression of power.

Strength in cheekbones appears in two areas: the base, the part of the cheekbone that forms the lower temple and socket of the eye and which can be prominent; and the knobs or points of the cheekbones that form the height of the cheeks below the eyes.

TYPES OF CHEEKBONES

A powerful cheekbone shows both a strong base and a strong bone. Katharine Hepburn is an excellent example of someone who has the ideally powerful cheekbone in a woman. This cheekbone shows good background, prestige, and power, but the woman who has such a

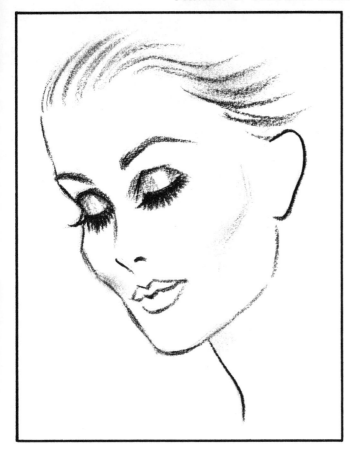

HIGH, SQUARE: STRONG BASE.
Great strength, power. Characteristic
of woman executives who need
strength to gain control.

cheekbone may be hard for others to agree with, and may be pretty much alone in her life.

Cheekbones that are high and round without a strong base are also indicative of someone who is hard to get along with—and who may not be a good mate because she is too willful and often exercises power without a firm purpose to back it up.

Cheekbones that are pointed and without a base are not considered good. They show someone who is shrewd, self-centered, and sometimes unkind.

High squarish cheekbones with a strong base are characteristic of women executives who need strength to control underlings. But such a woman may be alone in life because she finds it hard to discover a mate who is her equal in position and strength.

Flat cheekbones show someone who is easygoing, and not demanding. Such a person may not reach a high position in life, and is often self-employed. However, these are very easy people to work for. People like them, but they are not achievers.

If cheekbones are close to the nose and narrow, not too prominent, and are balanced with the nose, they give a high status without too much effort. If, however, the face is thin and the space between the cheekbones is narrow, the person may be unkind and selfish and difficult to deal with.

CHEEK MAKEUP

The purpose of blusher is to give a healthy glow to the face, but it can also be used to emphasize the cheekbones and give them more promi-

POINTED, NO BASE.
This indicates one who is shrewd and self-centered, perhaps often unkind.

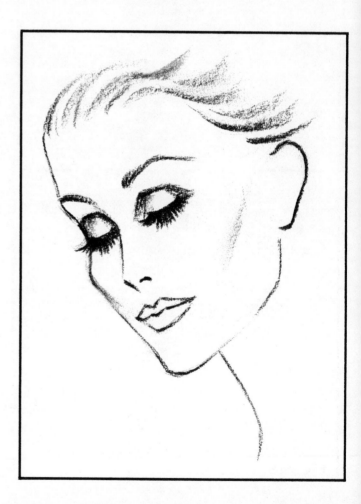

nence, or to modify too strong cheekbones.

The normal position of blusher is over the fatty part of the cheek, coming no closer to the nose than Points 46 and 47, and no lower on the face than the tip of the nose—or Points 58 and 59. Bring the blusher outward toward the temple but no higher than the outer tip of the eye.

If you want to thin the face or make the cheekbones more prominent, use a bright blusher at the upper part of the cheek starting at Points 46 and 47 and moving toward the temple, and a slightly darker blush below in the hollow of the cheeks, starting from Points 58 and 59 and moving toward Points 83 and 94. If you want to make the cheekbones less prominent, use the darker blusher from Points 47 and 46 along the line of the cheekbone to the temple.

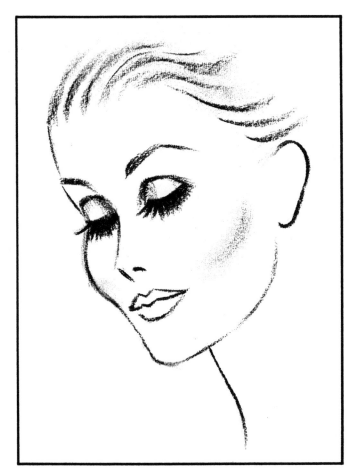

HIGH, ROUND, NO BASE.
May be willful, exercising power
without a firm purpose to back it up.

If for nighttime or for photography, you want to contour your cheekbones for dramatic effect, here is the easiest way to do it: Just pucker the lips, and you'll see the hollows of the cheeks clearly. The cheekbones will naturally stick out. Leave the *cheekbones* alone for now. Use a dark blush, preferably a brownish color, deep taupe or earth tone color, matte-finish (not frosted), and gently brush into the hollow area revealed by your lip pucker in a reverse (⌐) shape. Next, onto the part of the cheekbones that sticks out (not on top of the contour), put a lighter, brighter blush than you would ordinarily use. Or you can use a gloss on these cheek points for a nice interesting contrast. This is good for disco or other glamour makeup.

Selecting the right contour color should not be a problem. For most coloring, use a bronze. If you are very fair, use tawny. If you have dark skin or a very dark tan, use a deep earth color, brown or chocolate.

FLAT. Easygoing, undemanding—but not an achiever, often self-employed.

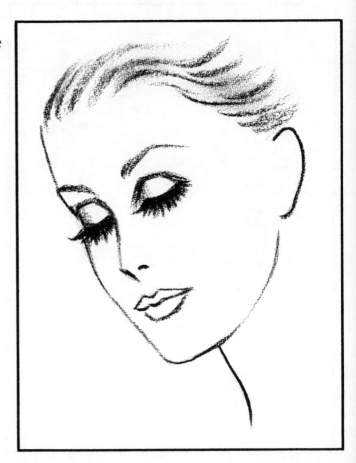

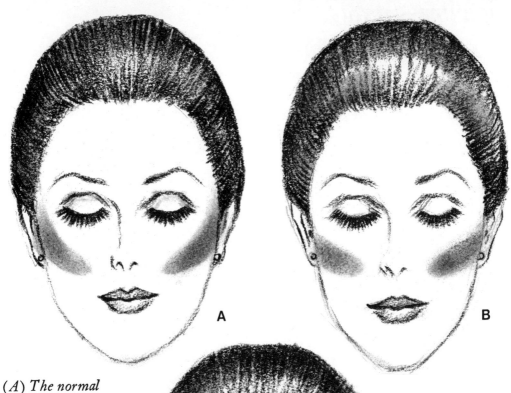

(A) The normal position of blusher is on the fatty part of the cheek. No closer to the nose than a point under the middle of the eye, no lower than the tip of the nose and fanned out toward the temples, but no higher than the outer tip of the eye.

(B) To widen a narrow face apply blusher almost horizontally along the line of the cheekbones toward the ears.

(C) To thin the face or make the cheekbones more prominent, use a bright blusher at the upper part of the cheek toward the temple and a slightly darker blush below in the hollows of the cheeks.

The Jawline—Status

THE JAW represents your status—your situation in life—and as you can see from the Map of the Face, the jawline is emphasized in the later years when the position you have attained in life is important to your well-being and comfort.

TYPES OF JAWS

The ideal jaw is firm and well molded, about equal in width to the forehead and not too short, rounded but slightly squared off so that it does not show weakness. This indicates a self-sufficient, accomplished, and successful person with balance, who can assure her own status and well-being in maturity.

If the jaw is round and smooth, it shows a good family, nice home, a pleasant disposition, and security and comfort in the later years.

The oval, tapering jaw, which is considered the "line of beauty," as it is part of the admired oval face, is not really good for old age. In youth this person does well, but there is usually weakness and dissatisfaction or ill health in late life.

If one has no jaw or a narrow weak jaw, it is again not favorable for health and long life. Often a receding jaw can be corrected with combined dentistry and plastic surgery.

If the jaw is very broad and very square, the person is self-centered and has no interest in the welfare of others and may be very stubborn and proud. It may lead to a high position but often to loneliness and distrust in late years.

A jaw that is so wide that its sides are visible from back of the head indicates an extremely domineering militant nature.

One should not try too much modeling with light and shade to change the shape of the jawline, as it can best be modified or strengthened by the way the hair is worn. However, there are some little tricks that do emphasize or deemphasize a problem jaw.

If the jaw is too wide or too square or sharp, a little blusher on the outer corners can make it seem less prominent.

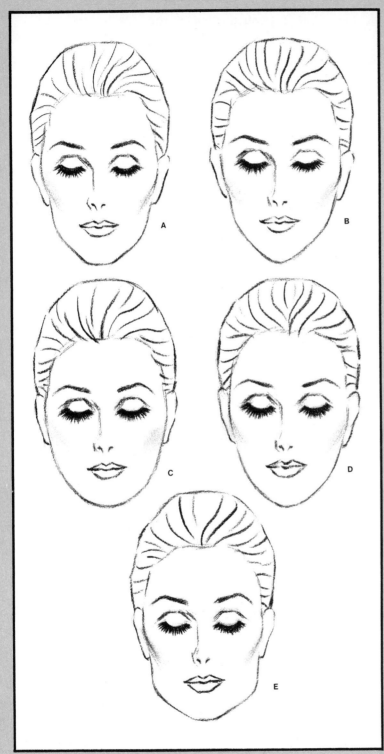

(A) FIRM, WELL-MOLDED.
Indicates an accomplished, successful person with balance. She can assure her own status and well-being in maturity.

(B) ROUND AND SMOOTH.
Good family, pleasant disposition, with security and comfort in later years.

(C) OVAL, TAPERING.
In youth, this person thrives but there is often weakness and dissatisfaction or ill health in later life.

(D) NARROW JAW.
Not favorable for health or long life. Often can be corrected with dentistry and plastic surgery.

(E) BROAD AND SQUARE.
Self-centered, stubborn, proud. High position but loneliness in late years. A little blusher on the outer corners can make it less prominent.

If the jaw (and chin) is weak and small, a popular trick of the theatre can be used to make it seem more definite. This involves using a slightly darker foundation on the throat than is used on the face and bringing the darker foundation up under the chin and lower jaw, where often the skin is paler because the sun does not strike there. This makes the whole lower face lighter so the jaw stands out.

If the jaw is strong and square, keeping a large volume of hair at jawline level can make it less outstanding. It should be considered that a strong jawline can be an asset to your looks, and perhaps should be made much of. A slight uneven jaw is more of a problem.

Like strong cheekbones, a strong jaw becomes more prominent in later years as the bony structure of the face matures and becomes more visible, and the jaw muscles are developed. Strong-jawed people are often highly articulate and become loquacious and even argumentative as they get along in life.

A basically fragile or weak jawline can diminish in later years, especially if teeth are lost or there is bone loss generally. Remember in your youth that calcium, phosphorous and vitamin E are the bone-protecting nutrients.

The Chin—Strength

THE CHIN is another "mountain" of the face and should be prominent. It represents our strength and as the Position Points of the sixties and seventies are on the chin, a strong chin indicates strength persisting into old age and hence a long life.

TYPES OF CHINS

The ideal chin has good form and is prominent; it should be round at the sides and squarish at the tip. This will lead to a strong healthy life and lusty offspring.

A pointed chin is connected with narrowness of mind and weakness in health, and suggests someone who is not too adaptable in personal relationships.

The chin that is rounded at the tip indicates a kind of weakness in character, as well as a long life—but one that will not be much fun.

The oval chin, though the standard for beauty, is somewhat weak and though its owner may be prosperous and strong during youth and middle-age, later in life the person tends to weaken and go downhill. It is not promising of children—ordinarily a source of strength in the later years.

Position Point 71, which dominates the chin, has much to do with how hard you must work in life and whether you will continue to work and be strong and active throughout your later years.

A dimple in the chin or a cleft chin indicates an adventuress, with the heart of a child, someone who never really matures or settles down.

There is not much you can do in making up your chin except to give it a touch of blusher to enliven your face, or, if it is weak, to strengthen it by using darker foundation on the throat (as for the jawline).

Cosmetic surgery, often including dental reconstruction, can do much to correct a problem chin—one that recedes too much or juts forward or is too prominent. This is costly and difficult plastic surgery because it involves removal or adjustment of bone and teeth, and often implants if the chin is to be built up. However, many women (and men) find the work worthwhile because our strength and courage are indeed judged by the chin.

The Undereye Area—Children

THE AREA UNDER THE EYE is one of the Seven Minor Features and its importance comes from its relationship to fertility. The Palace of Children is located here. Many women find this part of the face changes

(A) IDEAL CHIN.
Rounded at sides, squarish at tip. Leads to a strong healthy life and vigorous children.

(B) POINTED CHIN. Shows some lack of adaptability in personal relationships. May suggest weakness in health in later life.

(C) ROUNDED AT TIP.
A vacillating or weak character. Long life but not much vitality.

(D) OVAL CHIN.
Youth and middle-age are prosperous, but in old age this one weakens. Not promising for children.

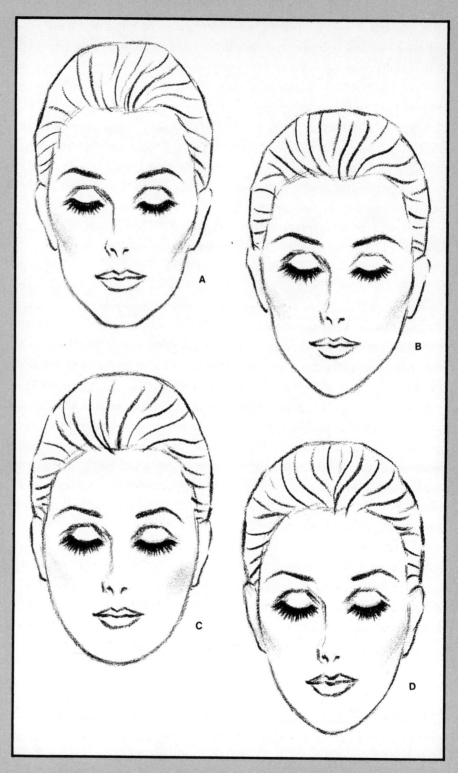

color during the various phases of the menstrual cycle, and in Chinese Face Reading the quality of this area determines whether you will be fortunate in your children—whether you will be fertile—and also influences your sexual desirability. This area tends to have a pleasant glow when a woman is pregnant.

The Chinese Face Readers call this area the "sleeping silkworm," because the pad of fat under the eye skin is curved and full like a silkworm in its cocoon.

TYPES OF UNDEREYE AREAS

There are four general types of formation in the undereye area:

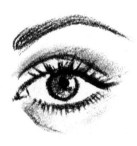

1. Very Puffy

This may be due to pads of fat under the eye or to water accumulation. In either case it is not considered an asset; it forebodes a weak constitution with little sexual stamina; one who may attract accidents. However, with bulging eyes, the characteristic improves somewhat—often this indicates an interesting character, one who has a good constitution, who meets dangerous situations easily, and enjoys games of chance.

VERY PUFFY. May be due to pads of fat or water accumulation. Forebodes a weak constitution with little sexual stamina. Mask with a natural-color foundation and a little undereye color cream at the tail of the eye to diminish the puff.

Excess puffiness under the eyes can be masked by using a slightly darker foundation on the undereye area to give less apparent fullness, and the use of a little undereye eye shadow at the tail of the eye to diminish the bulge. However, in the young, this puffiness, if slight, is often attractive, and children often have it. It looks youthful—in youth. The problem is that it can lead to bags under the eyes at a later date as gravity pulls the fat down and the skin under the eye stretches. Then, unfortunately, it makes one look dissolute, even if one isn't— and who wants to make an erroneous poor impression? Fortunately, these undereye bags can be corrected by cosmetic surgery rather simply —and should be if they become an "aging problem."

2. Slightly Puffy

With some undereye puffiness, you will have healthy children—and lots of them; you are sensuous and sexually desirable.

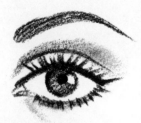

SLIGHTLY PUFFY.
Indicates one who is sensuous and sexually desirable— favorable for healthy children, high fertility.

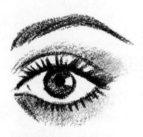

SUNKEN OR SHADOWED.
Not favorable for fertility and indicates a negative, pessimistic approach to life. Use a slightly lighter foundation under the eye, but blend it well into rest of face makeup. Bring blusher up over the corner of the eye to diminish circles and hollow effects.

3. Flat Undereye Area

This is nice to look at if the color is good, but it is not productive and a person with a flat smooth area here can expect to have only one or two children. It does give the impression of a woman who is beautiful and desirable, though in Face Reading it is a sign of being rather cold and materialistic. Often the person with this formation is narcissistic, and lets herself (or himself) be loved rather than loving.

4. Sunken or Shadowed

If the undereye area is hollow or is flat with shadows, it shows either poor metabolism or possible health problems developing around the reproductive system. People with sunken or shadowed eyes often cannot have children, or are not happy with their children, and have a negative, pessimistic approach to life.

Hollowness under the eye is not easily handled cosmetically. You can use a slightly lighter (this is *very slightly* lighter) foundation color under the eye to bring it out more, but blend it well into the rest of the cheek and eye makeup. Bringing the blusher up over the corner of the circle of the eye helps diminish both circles and sunken-eye effects. If the area is dark, as sometimes it becomes during the menstrual period, a foundation just a shade *darker* rather than lighter than your regular foundation can be used in a half-moon shape under the eye, brought down over the edge of the eye socket. Then apply your regular foundation over the edge of it and you will find it looks neither owl-eyed nor as dark as it otherwise would. If your shadows are chronic, and bother you, and if you wear glasses, the lower line of the rims should come below the socket of the eyebone to help conceal the shadows. Otherwise, follow the makeup directions for the deep-set eye (page 75) to attract attention away from the hollows or shadows and onto the pupils.

As undereye shadows, puffiness, hollows and so on are so often problems of health rather than heredity, it is a good idea to approach them from the health aspect. Consider what's wrong with your body, not only what's wrong with your face. The pads of fat under the eyes *are,* however, hereditary. And dark coloration under the eyes is a genetic characteristic in some ethnic groups.

On the positive side, shadows under the eyes are traditionally a sign of the sexually active and desirable person, and in matters of love are not as much a problem as they become in presenting yourself in public or in employment.

Tiny slanty lines going outward from the middle of the lower lash line toward the outer tip of the eye are normal in middle and older age, but when they are apparent in the young—especially a young man— they are a sign of one who is a poor risk for marriage. A union with such will be a problem and probably end in divorce, or he will otherwise make you miserable. He will not be a good father—may even desert his family. Guard against trusting your fate to such a heartbreaker.

The Philtrum—Productivity

THE PHILTRUM, the groove between the nose and the upper lip, is considered in Chinese Face Reading one of the Minor Features.

This feature is usually ignored in Western life. We don't even have a popular name for it. How often do you observe it? But in Chinese Face Reading it has a deep significance. It represents the life force. If the groove is deep, the person is very sensual; if well formed, the owner can have many children and a vital, long-lasting sex life. A flat or invisible groove or shallow groove shows someone who is not interested in sex either for its own sake or in order to have children.

The reason it represents sexuality is that the nose is considered the male and the mouth, the female. The philtrum connects the male and female representing intercourse between the sexes. The name philtrum has the same Greek root—*phil,* meaning loving—as "*phil*ter" (love potion) and "*phil*anderer" (male flirt), and the ancient Greeks also considered this groove an erotic feature.

Position Point 51 at the start of the groove is called the Center of Life—referring to this productive energy. As an age point, it represents the start of middle age. Many women find their sexual desires become stronger at this time (age fifty, when this feature and its Position Point are emphasized).

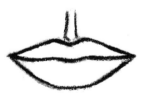

FLARED. Top is narrow, flares toward lips—promises productivity, sexual desirability and many offspring.

TYPES OF PHILTRUM

There are really only three types of philtrum that are important:

The top is narrow and flares toward the lips. This is the best type, promising productivity and a steady metabolism, sexual desirability and several children.

The top is wide but the groove gets narrower as it approaches the lips. This is not considered fertile and means less productivity—a single child or none.

If the groove is straight, you are not outstandingly productive, may have only one or two children, and will probably not have a superactive love life. However, if the groove is deep and meets perfectly the points of the upper lip, this is an asset for beauty and creates a more perfectly shaped mouth.

In all types, the depth as well as the shape is significant.

A flat, poorly shaped or disappearing groove—one that flattens or loses its formation near the lips—is not productive in business and will not attract a good clientele because we are basically attracted by people who are fertile—who have a strong life force—and are put off by those who lack this innate physical vitality.

A deep, well-shaped philtrum is helpful to anyone—salesperson, tour guide, waiter, receptionist—who must deal with the public in daily life.

There is no particular way to make up the philtrum—but it is involved in the shaping of the lips (see pp. 105–117) and it is an interesting feature to observe when you are forming relationships, business or personal. Observing the philtrum can help you understand the character of the persons you are dealing with and evaluate their productivity and lust for life. And also consider its meaning in your own face. That is, if you aren't going to be a very creative and productive person, what will you do with your life? You might get into work where you control other people's production—and marry a man who already has children. Children, of course, are denoted as well by other features in the face (the undereye area, for example), so you should examine your whole face, and those of others, for prospects in this respect.

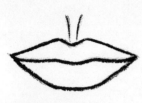

NARROWING. Top is wide, narrows toward lips—less productivity; not fertile—perhaps a single child or none.

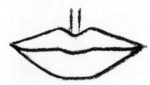

STRAIGHT. Not outstandingly productive, one or two children and not a superactive love life.

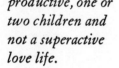

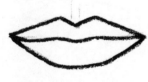

FLAT. When the philtrum is flat or loses its formation near the lips it is not productive and shows a weakening life force.

If the philtrum is deep and well-shaped, use your early years for fulfillment of the promise of this feature for your years after age fifty. You can be confident of your sexuality, your productivity, and life force.

Laugh Lines—Longevity

HERE IS ANOTHER FEATURE that we often give little consideration, but which is significant in Face Reading because it reveals health and long life. The cheek laugh lines reveal the life span. They separate the cheeks from the mouth area and so are related both to sensuality and power. Position Points 56 and 57 show the age at which the lines are most operative and at which time they often are present on the face even if you are not smiling.

TYPES OF LAUGH LINES

For good health and long life, the lines should be curved and long. If they are curved and of average length, you will live a good life but only an average life span.

If they are long and curve down and then out, you are a longevity "star"—you will have a particularly long life—and see five generations of your descendants.

If the laugh lines curve into the corners of the mouth, this indicates poor health in old age and possible destitution, even starvation, in one's last years.

If they are long and curve in below the mouth, it indicates a long life with loneliness at the end.

If they continue to curve out below the mouth, this gives vitality and much activity in the outside world in old age.

The laugh lines around the mouth often begin to be pronounced as one attains success in career. Women who have executive jobs and those who attain high positions in government often have pronounced laugh lines earlier than others. Women who are not in competitive situations often show these laugh lines only much later.

The lines are called Fa Ling and their Points—56 and 57—represent longevity.

Visible laugh lines are considered fortunate only after age forty. To make these lines less noticeable, use a light foundation or coverup cream to lighten them. Apply in the lines with fingertips and blend well. If these lines are very deep, they can be modified only by a total face-lifting. The maintenance of the teeth, particularly the back teeth, can prevent their becoming pronounced at too early an age. As deepening of these lines on the face is associated with an aging look, their relationship to longevity and good health is not surprising. And people who laugh a lot are said to live longer.

(A) CURVED, AVERAGE LENGTH.
Indicates a good life, but only an average life span.

(B) CURVED INTO MOUTH.
Poor health in old age and possible destitution in old age.

(C) LONG AND CURVED IN BELOW THE MOUTH.
A long life with loneliness at the end.

(D) LONG, CURVING OUT BELOW MOUTH.
Vitality and much activity in the outside world in old age.

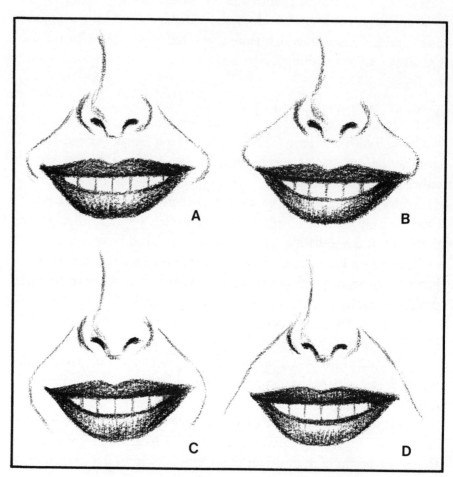

7. Balance Your Face with Your Hairdo and Accessories

YOUR HAIR—along with your brows and facial makeup, your neckwear and earrings—is your most useful asset in balancing your face and minimizing any too-prominent feature.

The Chinese Face Readers recognize that the condition of the hair and health are related, just as Westerners now do, and the character readings of hair are tied into health and vitality. Hair is also a status symbol; beautiful hair indicates a luxurious life.

HAIR TYPES

Hair that is of medium texture, not coarse or too fine, and of medium thickness and abundance (the Chinese strive always for balance!), that is silky and shiny, is considered ideal—the person is a doer, is in good health, has sound and creative ideas and reasonable ambition. This person will accomplish a great deal in middle life and have a happy old age.

Thin fine hair indicates a sensitive nature. The person will be artistic, involved in the arts as a writer or painter, or otherwise creative. But the person with this kind of hair may be too sensitive, perhaps timid and not aggressive enough to achieve all desired goals.

If hair is coarse, the person is usually temperamental. This person is active, aggressive, an achiever, often self-employed, or into sports or the military, because of the abundance of blood circulating to the head. This person is also tempestuous, with very strong opinions, and can be a powerful opponent.

If hair is very thick and abundant, there is no problem if the body is also large-boned and powerful. But in a small-boned person, the effect is not that positive. Somehow this person is forever in an unbalanced situation. Things are hard to accomplish and the promise of longevity is diminished.

If hair is very thin, the person is shrewd and possibly will seem old before her time. Something is perhaps not right in the system and life expectancy is not that great. If your hair is thin, look perhaps at your health and nutrition. But also remember that the quality of hair has a genetic factor. Perhaps you come from skinny-haired people.

Very curly hair indicates self-indulgence—the playgirl psychology. The curly-haired is likely to be irresponsible, perhaps promiscuous in sex, and generally not dependable or of a stable nature. The degree of curliness is important. Wavy hair is considered less frolicsome; slightly curly hair has only moderate tendencies to dalliance; but the real curlyhead is likely to be flirtatious and unreliable in love.

Graying Hair

If hair turns gray while one is very young, this is not a promising sign, and you will probably have a hard life ahead of you. But if you gray gradually in the middle years, this is an indicator of achievement, and to be gray in old age is considered a mark of honor.

If hair goes gray in youth and regains color later (in middle or old age), it may not mean trouble for you but it is unlucky for others. It can cause problems for your children, changing your destiny in some unfortunate way—as if your putting out new shoots in the later years weakens the main stem of the family tree.

Whatever your hair type, its shininess and good condition—as an indicator of your own basic health and vitality—is what is significant cosmetically.

Your hair style is changeable, usually very adaptable. You can work with it and your neckwear and earrings to modify the prominence or weakness of some features—the forehead, the nose, a prominent jaw, a weak chin, pronounced cheekbones, big ears. The purpose is "to balance your face."

The first thing, though, in this age of individuality, is whether you want to modify your face or emphasize an unusual feature. A high forehead, big ears, a prominent nose or chin, a square jaw can all be assets, so if you want to tie your hair back and go with your face as it is—or as you present it with artful makeup—fine! If you want to balance your face, here are suggestions.

1. Oval Face

If this is your face shape, you can wear any hair style comfortably—and a middle parting (if any) is your trademark because your face has the symmetry this equal division demands. Because you have something to show off, by beauty standards, you can brush your hair away from your face in simple lines, let it flow free, soften it with waves around the forehead, or tie it into a knot. Most any length will be becoming to you, granted your other features and ears are equally

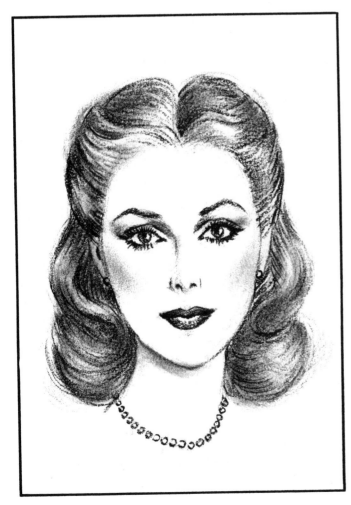

OVAL FACE. Most any hair length, any hairstyle is becoming to you. The middle parting is your trademark. Brush your hair away from your face to show off its symmetry.

ideal. Even an oval face can have a problem feature, so if you do have a prominent nose, small features with bushy hair, look under the specific problem for your answer.

2. Round Face

You need something off-center to break up the circle of your face. The usual solution is a high side part, lifted hair at the top of your head, but higher on the side away from the parting, which naturally brings more hair to one side anyway. It's a good idea to cover the tops of your ears, but to keep your hair off your neck (which often is short); choose unflipped waves (rather than tight curls); get plenty of volume high on your head and never go flat on top. Hair should dip a little on the forehead off center, again to break up the perfect circle. Avoid high round necklines, button earrings, choker or chunky necklaces. In-

ROUND FACE. An off-center parting breaks up the circle of your face—lift hair at the top of the head. Pendant earrings, V necklines become you.

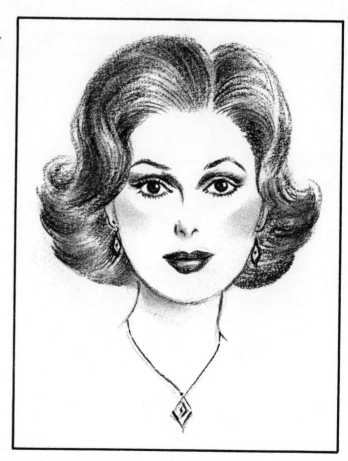

stead, V necklines or deep ovals; pendant or curved earrings. In neck-wear, choose pendants with an asymmetrical shape; scarves knotted low on your chest. In eyeglasses, choose somewhat square or straight-sided frames.

3. Square Face

Keep the parting high but slightly off-center, moving upward toward the crown rather than downward, and have softness around the fore-head (so the square line there is broken) and around the ears and back. Also becoming is fullness at the jawline, so that the hair swings over the square corners of the jaw, reducing the width in this area. Look for soft scooped or gentle V-necklines—not too high; rounded ear-rings of medium size or small gold hoops are becoming. *You* can wear rounded eyeglass frames.

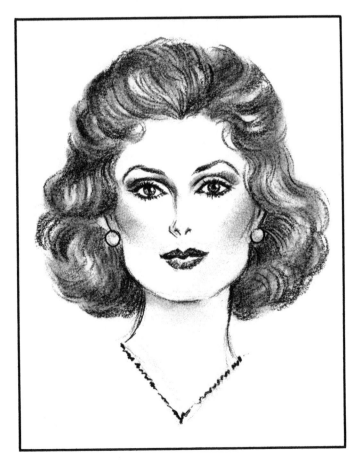

SQUARE FACE. Softness around the forehead, fullness at the jawline, gentle V or scooped necklines, rounded earrings modify the angles of the square face.

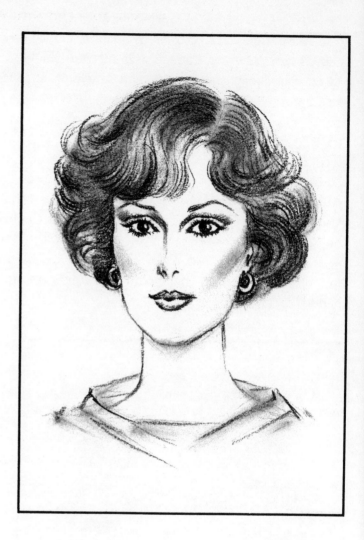

OBLONG FACE. Your face asks for softness in the hair—a side part with half bangs and full layers that keep the width at the cheekbone level. A cowl or boat neckline and medium-hoop earrings are becoming.

4. Oblong Face

Your face demands softness in the hair and some irregularity. A low side part with semi-bangs that break the length of the forehead, and fullness—or full layers that keep the width of your face at the cheekbone level. A straight-across neckline that carries the eye sideways at the breastbone is becoming. Or, if neck is long and thin, a cowl collar or shoulder-tied scarf. You can wear medium-size hoop earrings; eyeglass shape should provide width—glasses can be oval and fairly large —without coming too close at the nose. Keep the frame color light over the bridge of the nose so that you stretch the space between the eyes.

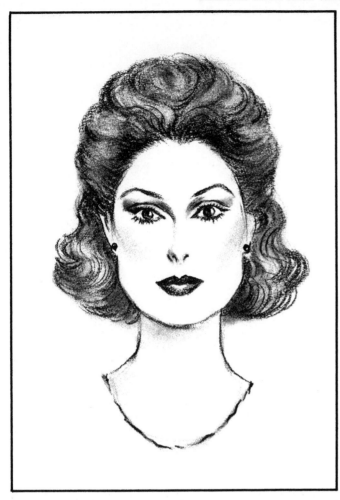

PEAR-SHAPED FACE. You need fullness below the jawline with lift (but not too high) and width at the forehead. Use small earrings and a deep scoop neckline or a wide V with pendant necklaces.

5. Pear-Shaped Face

With your wide Third Station, you need fullness just below the jawline so that the side hair swings over the jawbone and below. This works only if the neck is fairly long. If you have a short neck and have to wear short hair, start with a side part and a clear forehead, and lift the hair to give high width above forehead level (but not too much height). Curls help create volume; combs will hold the hair high. Use only small dot earrings. A wide deep scoop neckline or wide V makes your wide jaw less apparent. Wear interesting low-hanging pendant necklaces. Interesting eyeglasses can give important emphasis to the top of your face and help balance your jaw.

6. *Heart-Shaped Face*

This face is usually pert and pretty and appealing. Show off your Peach Blossom by keeping the forehead clean, with some lift in the forehead hair. You can bring the side hair softly down to cover some of the cheekbone width and create fullness behind and below the ear to give width to the small chin (but do not bring the hair forward to cover the jawbone). Pendant earrings help widen the chinline. A round neckline or a high neckline (unless the neck is short) also give you more chin.

7. *Diamond-Shaped Face*

Keep width and fullness at the forehead and below the ear and bring the hair close over your wide cheekbones. You do better, especially

HEART-SHAPED FACE. Show off your forehead peak by keeping forehead clear with soft lift in top hair. The hair may cover some cheekbone, with fullness behind and below the ear to give breadth to the small chin. Pendant earrings, a round neckline are becoming.

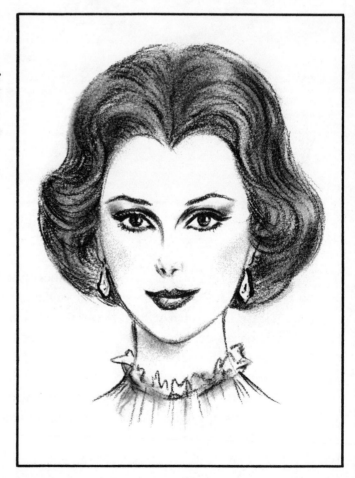

if the forehead is high, if you start from a high side part and swing the hair across the side of the forehead to be closest at the ears, but full below the ears. With this face, some softness and fullness is becoming. Pendant earrings only make your face appear longer. Use medium-size hoops, if any, but your hairdo will probably be more becoming if your ears are covered. Necklines and necklaces can be high; too long, they pull down your chin.

8. Triangular Face

Start with a high side part and bring some hair onto the forehead at both sides. If the ears are partly covered and there is some fullness behind them, it modifies your small chin. Avoid V necklines—you need deeply rounded or square necklines to give you more chin. Pendant

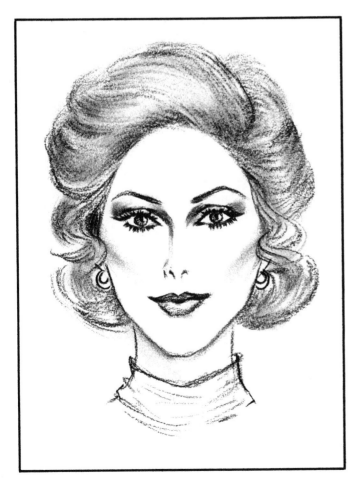

DIAMOND-SHAPED FACE. Keep width and fullness at the forehead and bring some hair over your wide cheekbones in tendrils or in a flat geometric shape, and have fullness below the ears to modify the sharp chin. Use medium hoop earrings, high necklines.

earrings suggest width in the lower part of your face. Eyeglass frames should be pale or pastel so that the emphasis is not too strong at the top of your face.

Fashions in hair change—so the solution to a problem feature that works one year may not work the next.

· Most women with irregular features or prominent noses or chins or high or too-wide foreheads needs some softness about the face.

· A flat-top hairdo is usually not becoming to those with round or square faces (the Stations are too short).

TRIANGULAR FACE. A high side part and some hair on the forehead at both sides cuts the high and wide forehead. Keep the ears only partly covered with some fullness behind them to modify your small chin. Round or square necklines, pendant earrings balance this face.

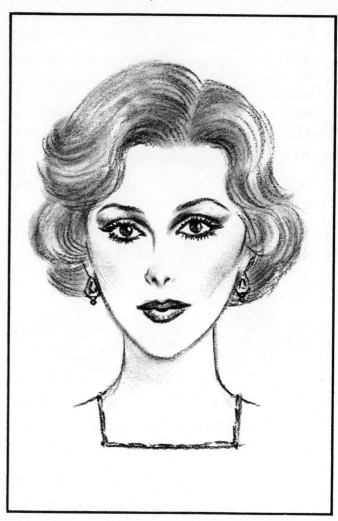

- A middle part is unbecoming to an oblong face or a diamond face—the face is too long for this symmetrical division.

- Thick bangs should be avoided by those with low foreheads, pear-shaped faces, triangular faces (you look top-heavy).

- Very short or severe hairdos should be avoided by those with square or oblong faces or very large faces.

- If features are small, you have to watch out for too-full hair.

- If the face is large (it is considered good fortune to have a large face, however!), avoid too much volume as well as too-close hairdos. You need a happy medium, with some fullness but not too much length.

- If the nose is prominent, you can take a tip from Nefertiti, the Egyptian queen, who balanced her nose with height at the back of the crown, although this may become too dramatic and too severe a look for everyday. Another solution is fullness at the top front, to soften but not completely cover the forehead. Flat-top hairdos are to be avoided. Give your face all the width you can, but cover your ears and have some fullness below the ears.

- For a prominent chin, some forehead fullness with length over the ears and the sides of the jaw tapering to the nape can be becoming.

- Where you put the parting in the hair is important for most face balancing. A middle parting or very low side part is usually becoming. For most faces, other than the oval, a high side part will be most flattering.

- If you have a prominent Second Station (middle face), keep the hair off the forehead and wear hair longer than the chin.

- If you have a prominent First Station (forehead), cover your hairline, whether with short curls or sideswept bangs.

- If your Third Station (lower face) is prominent, keep your hair above jaw length and your forehead clear, and get height on top.

- If your face and features are small, keep hair close to head.

- If face and features are large, use your hair to create volume.

BALANCE YOUR FACE WITH YOUR
EYEGLASS FRAMES

If contact lenses work for you, and you can afford them, and you need day-long and night-vision correction, they're a beauty asset. They give your eyes extra glow and they don't create beauty problems. However, you probably still will need a pair of glasses, and even those who don't need vision correction often wear sunglasses. You can make eyeglasses an asset, too, because they can, well chosen, help balance your face.

If you wear glasses for vision correction, it's best to stay away from gimmicky frames—frames with odd shapes, very dark, or in bright colors—unless you can afford several pairs. There are exceptions. Your particular face may need just such an attention getter, and if it works for you, fine.

Otherwise, you can use frames to enhance your face. The secret is to follow the natural browline with the top of the frame. The frame should not let the brow show above or below.

- If your face is oblong or squarish, don't emphasize the squareness with a square frame. Choose one that is round or oval.
- If your face is round, choose a square frame or one that has straight lines across the top and bottom.
- Avoid frames that are very dark. Warm browns, roses, rusts, ambers flatter a pale or sallow skin; if your face is florid, choose cool colors— blues, greens, grays.
- If features are small or face is small, avoid frames that are large and overpowering; if your face is large, again don't get enormous glasses that make it overwhelming, but look for large frames in proportion to your face.
- If eyes are wide-set, you can choose a darker bridge to bring the eyes closer together.
- If eyes are close-set or deep-set or small, choose a frame that is lighter over the bridge.
- If nose is long, choose a darker, heavier bridge and one that is low-set.
- If nose is short or wide, choose a high or medium-set pale bridge.

8. Cosmetic Surgery— Can It Change Your Fate?

CERTAINLY, if you are unhappy with a feature or features, and cosmetic surgery can help you achieve what you want—and if you can afford it—it can have a positive effect, at least psychologically. With the explosion of cosmetic surgery, prices are no longer out of line and experienced surgeons are doing fine work. Baggy eyes are coming out of hiding; unfortunate noses are being remodeled, chins built up, underchin wattles excised, and whole faces lifted. It won't change your fate, but it can change your attitude— and that can change your fortune.

To answer the obvious question, the Position Points remain the same even if you have moved your laugh lines an inch up your cheeks with a face lift. You'll still be a swinger, even if you have your crow's feet smoothed. The suspending needle between your brows may be erased, but its indications will stay with you. Even if your forehead lines are modified, their good luck stays in your life. A round nose, however, unless it is bulbous, seems a shame to sacrifice.

One thing to remember when you have cosmetic surgery—and any ethical cosmetic surgeon will tell you this—is that you cannot always have the nose of your dreams even with surgery. The feature has to remain in harmony with your face—and unless *all* your bone structure is to be remodeled, you may, for example, come out with a better nose, but not a perfect nose.

Bear in mind, too, that not *all* cosmetic surgery produces the wanted results; sometimes there are side effects (poor breathing, trouble closing your eyes); removing wattles does leave a scar under the chin. Sometimes there are undesirable psychological effects; neurotic reactions may develop; you may not recognize your new face. And a face lift is not forever; it may take ten years off your looks, but time puts it right back on, and then you need another remodeling.

In China, age has traditionally been revered. The goal of a long life is a major one. In Western youth-oriented society, looking young as well as being young is valued. Looking old can be a handicap.

If a face lifting can give you ten more good years—or better years —or an eye job can open up your face or a nose bob make you more confident, it certainly can be an investment in happiness.

Perhaps, though, by understanding the meaning of your features, you'll feel happier with them as they are.